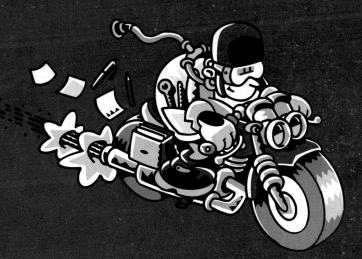

Surgery

Series editor
Wilfred Yeo
BMedSci, MB, ChB, MD, MRCP
Senior Lecturer in Medicine,
Medicine/Clinical
Pharmacology and
Therapeutics,
University of
Sheffield

Faculty advisor
Helen Sweetland
MB, ChB, MD, FRCS
Senior Lecturer and
Consultant Surgeon,
University Department
of Surgery,
University of Wales
College of Medicine,
Cardiff

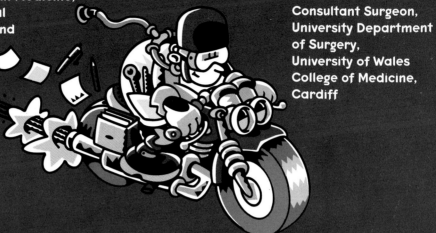

Surgery

Helen Sweetland
MB, ChB, MD, FRCS
Senior Lecturer and
Consultant Surgeon,
University Department of
Surgery,
University of Wales College of
Medicine,
Cardiff

James Cook
MB, ChB, FRCS(Ed)
Surgical Registrar
Cheltenham General
Hospital
Cheltenham

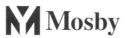 Mosby

London Edinburgh New York Philadelphia Sydney Toronto

Editor	Louise Crowe
Project Manager	Lindy van den Berghe
Designer	Greg Smith
Layout	Kate Walshaw
Illustration Management	Mick Ruddy
Illustrator	Marion Tasker
Cover Design	Greg Smith
Index	Janine Ross

ISBN 0 7234 3154 X

Copyright © Harcourt Publishers Limited 1999.

Published in 1999 by Mosby, an imprint of Harcourt Publishers Limited.

Text set in Crash Course–VAG Light; captions in Crash Course–VAG Thin.

Cataloguing in Publication Data
Catalogue records for this book are available from the British Library and the US Library of Congress.

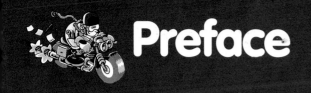

Preface

Patients present to doctors with symptoms rather than diagnoses. Medical students are often amazed at the speed at which doctors can make a diagnosis, but it comes from the experience of seeing a wide variety of patients. As you spend time on surgical attachments you will see that surgeons spend some time operating, but a considerable period of time talking and examining patients to make a diagnosis.

The first part of this book deals with common presentations to a surgical outpatient clinic or as emergencies to surgical house officers. It will help you to ask relevant questions and plan investigations in a systematic way. The rest of the book gives background information on all the conditions mentioned.

This book should be helpful to students starting their first surgical attachment to give an overview of the topic and it can also be used later as a revision book. I hope that it will stimulate an interest in surgery so that you will want to read more about some of the topics.

Surgery is a fascinating subject that brings anatomy to life. It is a dynamic specialty and this book should help you to get involved and enjoy surgery.

Helen Sweetland

Many, if not most, undergraduate text books in clinical specialties, provide the student with comprehensive information about specific conditions. It is often left to the student, however, to determine how this information can be extracted in the clinical setting to establish the diagnosis. Often the diagnosis can be clinched by asking just a few vital questions and performing the right investigation rather than a whole barrage of tests. (Just look at your consultants' outpatient notes for an example of this!)

Crash Course Surgery will be useful to both junior clinical students and those of you about to enter your first years as a doctor, by giving a helping hand in targetting your enquiries and investigations to gain more information for less effort. It also provides background information on conditions organized by organ system as well as management suggestions once the diagnosis has been established.

Surgery is a rewarding subject and I hope this book helps you get the most out your time in this specialty.

James Cook

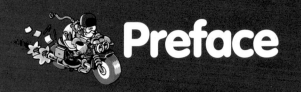

Preface

So you have an exam in medicine and you don't know where to start? The answer is easy—start with *Crash Course*. Medicine is fun to learn if you can bring it to life with patients who need their problems solving. Conventional medical textbooks are written back-to-front, starting with the diagnosis and then describing the disease. This is because medicine evolved by careful observations and descriptions of individual diseases for which, until this century, there was no treatment. Modern medicine is about problem solving, learning methods to find the right path through the differential diagnosis, and offering treatment promptly.

This series of books has been designed to help you solve common medical problems by starting with the patient and extracting the salient points in the history, examination, and investigations. Part II gives you essential information on the physical examination and investigations as seen through the eyes of practising doctors in their specialty. Once the diagnosis is made, you can refer to Part III to confirm that the diagnosis is correct and get advice regarding treatment.

Throughout the series we have included informative diagrams and hints and tips boxes to simplify your learning. The books are meant as revision tools, but are comprehensive, accurate, and well balanced and should enable you to learn each subject well. To check that you did learn something from the book (rather than just flashing it in front of your eyes!), we have added a self-assessment section in the usual format of most medical exams—multiple-choice and short-answer questions (with answers), and patient management problems for self-directed learning. Good luck!

Wilf Yeo
Series Editor (Clinical)

Contents

Contents

Contents

Contents

Contents

Acknowledgements

For loan of slides for illustrations: from University Hospital of Wales, Cardiff—Mr MCA Puntis for Fig. 8.2 (endoscopic retrograde cholangiopancreatogram); Mr Webster for Fig 16.1a (intravenous urogram); Dr C Evans for Fig. 16.1b (intravenous urogram); Mr. C. Darby for Fig. 36.1 (arteriogram); and from Kings Mill Centre for Health Care Sources—Miss J Patterson for Fig. 25.2 (corkscrew oesophagus).

To all those who have encouraged and
supported me in my surgical career.

HS

To Gillian, Frazer and Kirsty.

JC

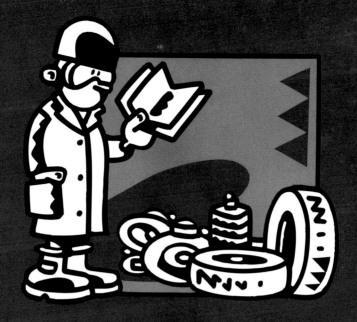

THE PATIENT PRESENTS WITH

1. Acute Abdominal Pain

Acute abdominal pain is the most common presenting surgical emergency. The main aim of the clinician seeing a patient who has acute abdominal pain is to recognize the serious causes from the not so serious. Many patients are admitted with abdominal pain, but only 20% will need any surgical intervention to speed their recovery. The rest may need investigations to find out the cause of the pain, but there is a group of patients who are labelled as having 'non-specific abdominal pain (NSAP) ? cause'.

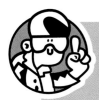

Medical conditions mimicking acute abdomen include:
- ○ **Lower lobe pneumonia**
- ○ **Inferior myocardial infarction**
- ○ **Hypercalcaemia**
- ○ **Hyperglycaemia**

DIFFERENTIAL DIAGNOSIS OF ACUTE ABDOMINAL PAIN

There are many different diagnoses for acute abdominal pain and they can be categorized by site as follows:
- Right upper quadrant—gall bladder disease.
- Epigastrium—peptic ulcer, peptic perforation, pancreatitis.
- Left upper quadrant—splenic rupture.
- Umbilical—gastroenteritis, small bowel obstruction, early appendicitis, mesenteric ischaemia.
- Right or left flank—renal colic, pyelonephritis, leaking aortic aneurysm.
- Suprapubic—cystitis, acute urinary retention, pelvic appendicitis.
- Right iliac fossa—mesenteric adenitis, appendicitis, Crohn's disease of the terminal ileum, carcinoma of the caecum, ovarian cyst, salpingitis, ectopic pregnancy.
- Left iliac fossa—diverticulitis, carcinoma of the sigmoid colon, ulcerative colitis, constipation, ovarian cyst, salpingitis, ectopic pregnancy.
- Groin—irreducible hernia.

HISTORY TO FOCUS ON THE DIFFERENTIAL DIAGNOSIS OF ACUTE ABDOMINAL PAIN

A full and thorough history of abdominal pain will be the most useful guide to establishing a likely cause.

Site

Many abdominal pains change site as the disease progresses (Fig. 1.1). The abdominal viscera have no somatic sensation so the pain is often felt initially in the dermatome (usually indicated in the midline) that is related to the embryological development of the gut. It may be:
- Epigastric—indicating foregut pathology.
- Central—indicating midgut pathology.
- Suprapubic—indicating hindgut pathology.

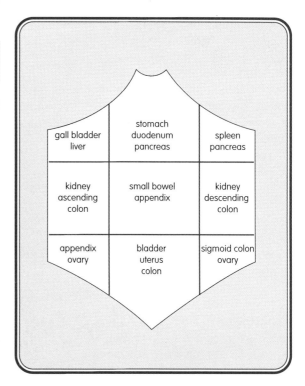

Fig. 1.1 Organs causing pain in the different abdominal regions.

This is often an important start to finding the cause.

As inflammation progresses the parietal peritoneum overlying the organ becomes inflamed and this causes a localized pain in that area, as listed in the differential diagnosis. For example in acute appendicitis the pain is initially vague and in the central abdomen and then moves to the right iliac fossa when the peritoneum becomes inflamed.

Onset
Is the pain sudden in onset or more insidious?
- An inflammatory condition tends to produce a gradual onset of pain that increases as the inflammatory reaction progresses.
- A ruptured viscus typically causes a sudden onset of pain.
- Smooth muscle colic, as in bowel obstruction or ureteric colic, has a rapid onset
- Hormonally induced smooth muscle colic, such as biliary colic, has a slow onset because the hormone (in this case cholecystokinin) only gradually increases in concentration.

Severity
Ask the patient to grade the pain on a scale of 1 to 10.

Renal colic is said to be one of the worst pains. Many women say that it is worse than childbirth.

Nature
The pain may be described in many terms by the patient. The more common include:
- Aching—a dull pain that is often poorly localized.
- Burning—this may be used to describe symptoms of a peptic ulcer (see Chapter 2).
- Stabbing—a short sharp sudden pain, as may be felt with ureteric colic. (Note, however, that the pain associated with a stabbing is often described as burning in nature.)
- Gripping—often associated with smooth muscle spasm as seen in bowel obstruction. The patient will often describe it with a wringing motion of their hands (as if wringing out a cloth).

Progression
How has the pain changed over time?
- It may be constant—seen in peptic ulcer
- It may be colicky—each sharp pain may last seconds (bowel), minutes (ureteric) or tens of minutes (gall bladder).

- It may change character completely. Appendicitis starts as a colicky central abdominal pain that then localizes to the right iliac fossa as a sharp pain that is worse on movement.

Radiation
The pain may seem to 'go through' to another part of the body. Often this can be quite revealing as to the cause of the pain. Good examples of radiation and causative organs are:
- Back—pancreas and other retroperitoneal structures.
- Shoulder tip—referred diaphragmatic pain (C4 dermatome—phrenic nerve).
- Scapula—gall bladder.
- Sacroiliac region—ovary.
- Loin to groin—typical description of ureteric colic.

Cessation
Does the pain go away slowly or quickly?
- Colicky pains, such as ureteric colic or bowel colic, usually have an abrupt ending.
- Inflammatory pain resolves slowly.
- Gall bladder colic also resolves slowly.

Exacerbating and relieving factors
Abdominal pathology causing inflammation of the peritoneum causes pain on movement so the patient lies still.

Ureteric colic is neither exacerbated nor relieved with movement and patients roll around trying to get comfortable.

Food may relieve or exacerbate the pain (see Chapter 2).

Associated symptoms
These may include:
- Nausea and vomiting (see Chapter 3).
- Constipation—there is a sudden onset of constipation, especially absolute constipation (where neither faeces nor flatus is passed) associated with vomiting faeculent fluid and colicky abdominal pain in bowel obstruction. These same features in the absence of colicky pain may be seen in ileus.
- Anorexia—a sudden onset of loss of appetite can be associated with any intra-abdominal pathology and should always be investigated further.
- Rectal bleeding (see Chapter 6).
- Fever and malaise—associated with inflammatory and infective conditions.

- Menstrual irregularity—a gynaecological history should be obtained from all women who have abdominal pain as menstrual irregularity may indicate ectopic pregnancy or chronic salpingitis.

EXAMINATION OF PATIENTS WHO HAVE ACUTE ABDOMINAL PAIN

General appearance
The patient's general appearance can give clues to the underlying pathology:
- Sweating—may be associated with a pyrexia and is also seen in hypotension due to intra-abdominal bleeding or sequestration of fluid (as seen in peritonitis or pancreatitis).
- Pallor—the patient may be anaemic due to bleeding, but may also be 'peripherally shutdown' in hypotensive states.
- Peritonitic facies—pale sweaty face with sunken eyes and a grey complexion.

Attitude in bed
The clinician's first impression of the patient in bed may suggest the diagnosis. The patient may be:
- Restless—typically seen in colic (either of the gastrointestinal tract or ureteric colic).
- Still—with movement exacerbating pain (as in peritonitis).
- Drawing up his or her knees—this position is often associated with severe peritonitis.
- Sitting forward—this lifts retroperitoneal structures away from the spine so may be a feature of the patient who has pancreatitis.

Temperature
The patient's temperature may be:
- Low—in states of shock such as severe peritonitis or pancreatitis.
- Increased—if the patient has infective pathology, especially pyelonephritis.

Vital signs
Check the following:
- Blood pressure—may be low in cases of haemorrhage or more frequently in peritonitis, where large volumes of fluid can be 'lost' in the gut and there is no intake of fluid.
- Pulse—a rapid pulse also reflects hypovolaemia (usually before a drop in blood pressure) and the pulse may be increased in infective conditions.
- Respiration—shallow, rapid breaths are associated with generalized peritonitis.

Abdominal examination
Inspection
The abdomen should be carefully inspected for:
- Scars—there may be adhesions inside the abdomen from previous surgery causing obstruction. The previous operation may have been for malignant disease, making a diagnosis of recurrent tumour high on the list of differential diagnoses.
- Masses—large masses may be visible.
- Movement—the patient who has peritonitis breathes shallowly and minimizes abdominal movement.
- Pulsatility—epigastric pulsation can be seen in the normal resting abdomen, but very prominent pulsations may be associated with an aortic aneurysm.
- Hernias—check the hernial orifices because irreducible hernias can cause small bowel obstruction.

Palpation
Gentle palpation is very important for gaining useful information. Starting with deep palpation will cause the patient to voluntarily tense his or her abdominal muscles to avoid further discomfort. Examination may demonstrate masses and tenderness. Signs of peritoneal inflammation include:
- Rigid abdomen—the abdominal muscles are contracted involuntarily. This is a sign of generalized peritonitis.
- Guarding—a localized area of involuntary muscle spasm indicating underlying peritoneal irritation.
- Rebound tenderness—the release of pressure on the peritoneum causes irritation as the peritoneum rubs against the inflamed organ.

Percussion
Solid or fluid-filled masses and gas-filled structures can be distinguished by percussion. Percussion is also probably the best test for rebound tenderness and is far more gentle than pressing the hand into the abdomen and pulling away sharply.

Auscultation
Bowel sounds are absent in ileus due to peritonitis. Loud high-pitched bowel sounds are heard in bowel obstruction.

Rectal and vaginal examination

These form an essential part of the abdominal examination. Rectal examination may reveal:

- Tenderness of the appendix in a pelvic appendicitis.
- Boggy swelling of a pelvic abscess.
- A large prostate gland causing urinary retention.
- An obstructing rectal carcinoma.

Vaginal examination may reveal:

- Vaginal discharge in salpingitis.
- Cervical tenderness or excitation in salpingitis or ectopic pregnancy.

- Retained tampon causing toxic shock.
- Pelvic mass such as ovarian cyst, pelvic abscess or fibroid uterus.

INVESTIGATION OF PATIENTS WHO HAVE ACUTE ABDOMINAL PAIN

An algorithm for the investigation and diagnosis of acute abdominal pain is given in Fig. 1.2.

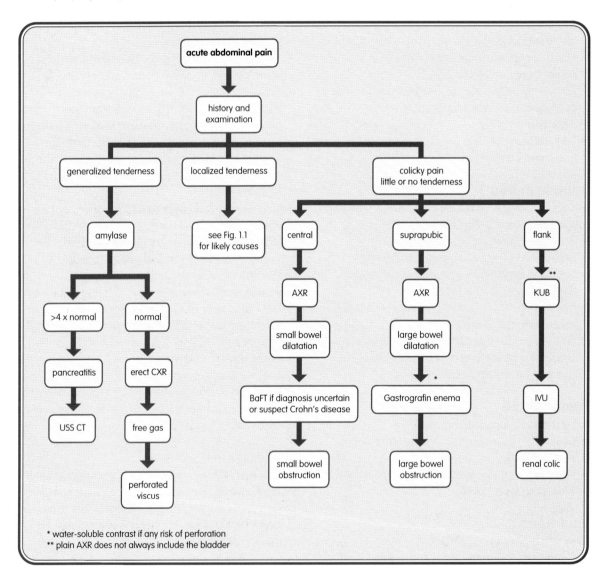

* water-soluble contrast if any risk of perforation
** plain AXR does not always include the bladder

Fig. 1.2 Investigation and diagnosis of acute abdominal pain (AXR, abdominal radiography; BaFT, barium follow-through; CT, computed tomography; CXR, chest radiography; KUB, kidneys, ureter, and bladder radiography; IVU, intravenous urography; USS, ultrasound scan.)

Blood tests
Full blood count
Findings may include:
- Low haemoglobin in cases of gastrointestinal haemorrhage or chronic blood loss.
- High haemoglobin in patients who are severely dehydrated and have peritonitis or pancreatitis.
- Increased white cell count in infective conditions.

Urea and electrolytes
These are measured to assess renal function and reveal dehydration. The potassium level is important if anaesthesia is required for a surgical operation.

Liver function tests
Liver function may be deranged as a result of diseases of the gall bladder and biliary tree (see Chapter 8)

Amylase
This is primarily measured to diagnose pancreatitis. Typically the amylase level will be increased more than four times the upper limit of normal (normal ranges vary between hospitals). Other conditions such as a perforated duodenal ulcer or ischaemic bowel may also give rise to a high amylase level, so the test should not be used alone to diagnose pancreatitis.

Arterial blood gases
Acidosis may be a sign of severe sepsis or ischaemic bowel.

Group and save
Blood should be sent for a group and save pending the full blood count and if there is any possibility that the patient will be having an operation.

Urine
Urine should be tested with a dipstick for the presence of:
- Red cells—seen in ureteric colic and infection.
- White cells—seen in infection.
- Nitrites—a breakdown product of urea seen in infection.

If any of these are present in the urine then urine should be sent for urgent microscopy and culture.

All premenopausal women who could be pregnant should have a pregnancy test.

Radiography
Chest radiography
An erect chest radiograph may show:
- Subphrenic free gas—indicating a perforation of a hollow viscus.
- Subphrenic bubbles—may be seen in cases of a subphrenic abscess.
- Lower lobe pneumonia—may cause hypochondrial pain.

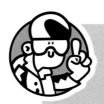

Approximately 30% of acute perforations are not evident on an erect chest radiograph.

Abdominal radiography
Plain abdominal radiography may show:
- Dilated loops of bowel associated with an obstruction—can give some idea about the level of obstruction.
- Free gas—may be seen outside the lumen of the bowel.
- Thick-walled inflamed bowel—is suggested by the presence of a widened space between adjacent loops of bowel.
- Stones may be seen—over 90% of kidney stones and less than 10% of gallstones are visible on a plain film.
- Gas in the biliary tree—seen in gallstone ileus with a cholecystoduodenal fistula.

Ultrasonography
This may demonstrate:
- Gallstones, dilated common bile duct, abnormal gall bladder.
- Inflamed pancreas or pseudocyst.
- Liver metastases or cysts.
- Aortic aneurysm.
- Large bladder.
- Dilated pelvicalyceal system in ureteric obstruction.
- Ovarian cysts.
- Hydro- or pyosalpinx.
- Abdominal or pelvic collections.
- Masses.

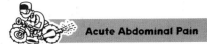

Computed tomography

This is better for demonstrating retroperitoneal structures such as the pancreas. It also gives better definition of masses.

Limited barium or Gastrografin enema

If the plain abdominal film shows dilated large bowel and an empty rectum a single contrast barium enema can reveal any mechanical obstruction. If there is any possibility of perforation a water-soluble contrast should be used.

Laparotomy

An ill patient showing signs of peritonism should undergo laparotomy to treat the underlying cause.

Occasionally a diagnosis of pancreatitis is made at laparotomy, but this is preferable to missing a perforated duodenal ulcer or colon.

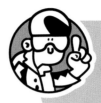

Beware of a silent perforation in the elderly and patients on corticosteroids.

Laparoscopy

This is used increasingly to diagnose the cause of lower abdominal pain in women.

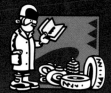

2. Dyspepsia

Dyspepsia describes an epigastric discomfort felt in many conditions. It is generally a symptom of upper gastrointestinal disease, but other conditions can produce similar symptoms. Patients may describe the symptoms of 'heartburn' (a retrosternal discomfort) or 'waterbrash' (the feeling of acid coming up into the throat).

DIFFERENTIAL DIAGNOSIS OF DYSPEPSIA

The differential diagnosis of dyspepsia includes:
- Duodenal ulcer.
- Gastric ulcer and gastritis.
- Gastric cancer.
- Hiatus hernia, oesophagitis, and gastro-oesophageal reflux disease.
- Gallstone disease.
- Non-ulcer dyspepsia.
- Irritable bowel syndrome.

HISTORY TO FOCUS ON THE DIFFERENTIAL DIAGNOSIS OF DYSPEPSIA

Site of pain

Dyspepsia is concerned with the upper gastrointestinal tract and therefore tends to produce epigastric pain, but there may be pain elsewhere:
- Retrosternal pain is suggestive of gastro-oesophageal reflux and oesophagitis.
- Gall bladder pain is typically referred through to the tip of the right scapula (note that pain at the tip of the shoulder is usually diaphragmatic pain, i.e. C4).

Characteristics of pain

Most dyspepsia is described as a 'burning pain', but variations in the character of pain are typical of different conditions:
- The pain of oesophagitis may be described as a tightness or crushing pain and can be confused with myocardial pain.

- Biliary colic is a severe pain that usually starts after eating fatty food and slowly builds up to constant pain lasting over 20 min with slow relief of pain.

Oesophageal pain may mimic angina. Both may be relieved by glyceryl trinitrate. Always check an electrocardiogram if in any doubt.

Exacerbating and relieving factors

Food can either exacerbate or relieve dyspepsia depending upon the condition:
- Gastric ulcer pain is typically made worse by food.
- Duodenal ulcer pain is relieved by food and exacerbated by starvation so the patient may complain of pain at night.

Certain types of food may exacerbate the pain:
- Fatty food typically produces biliary colic.
- Hot and spicy foods exacerbate the pain of gastric and duodenal ulcers.
- Milky foods help relieve the symptoms of peptic ulcer, but its fat content can worsen the pain of biliary colic.

Gastro-oesophageal reflux and oesophagitis are made worse when the patient lies down or bends over. Obesity exacerbates the problem.

Associated symptoms

Symptoms associated with dyspepsia include:
- Vomiting and nausea.
- Jaundice.
- Bloating.
- Weight loss.

Nausea is common with most causes of dyspepsia. Vomiting may be associated with a gastric outflow obstruction associated with duodenal ulcer or gastric malignancy (see Chapter 3). Jaundice is associated with biliary disease (see Chapter 8). Marked weight loss is usually associated with gastric malignancy. Irritable bowel syndrome often presents with the triad of colicky pain, abdominal bloating and alternating bowel habit. It is a diagnosis of exclusion, but a triad of such symptoms may alert the clinician to the possibility of this diagnosis at an early stage.

Drugs

A careful drug history (including alcohol and cigarettes) should be obtained:
- Non-steroidal anti-inflammatory drugs and corticosteroids are well known causes of peptic ulceration.
- Cigarette smoking is associated with an increased incidence of peptic ulcer.
- Excessive alcohol intake is a risk factor for peptic ulcer and can, in acute ingestion, cause severe gastritis.

EXAMINATION OF PATIENTS WHO HAVE DYSPEPSIA

General examination

General examination of the patient should look for:
- Signs of recent weight loss—suggesting possible malignant underlying disease.
- Anaemia in the absence of any overt blood loss —may indicate an occult source of blood loss such as a chronic ulcer or malignancy.
- Jaundice.
- Lymphadenopathy, especially in the left supraclavicular fossa (Virchow's node)—may indicate upper gastrointestinal malignancy.

Abdominal examination

The abdomen should be examined carefully, noting areas of tenderness and any palpable masses (see Chapter 1).

INVESTIGATION OF PATIENTS WHO HAVE DYSPEPSIA

An algorithm for the investigation and diagnosis of dyspepsia is given in Fig. 2.1.

Weight

The patient should be weighed and his or her weight compared with any previous recorded weight or the patient's estimate of his or her weight.

Blood tests

These may include:
- A full blood count—to check for anaemia (especially chronic iron deficiency).
- Urea and electrolytes—if there is a history of vomiting (see Chapter 3).
- Liver function tests—may show derangement in the presence of gallstone disease (see Chapter 8).

Barium meal

Contrast studies of the stomach can reveal many pathologies, including:
- Hiatus hernia.
- Reflux—can be demonstrated with fluoroscopic screening.
- Large gastric ulcers and tumours.
- Scarring of the duodenum.

Endoscopy

This is a better investigation for dyspepsia. With the exception of active reflux, all of the above may be seen at endoscopy and it is possible to visualize and biopsy the mucosal abnormalities to look for:
- Barrett's oesophagus.
- Malignant change in gastric ulcers (5–10% will be malignant).
- *Helicobacter pylori*.

Ultrasonography

This is primarily used for assessing the biliary tree, to look for gallstones, any dilatation of the biliary tree, and gallbladder wall thickness, indicating the presence or not of inflammation.

Manometry and pH monitoring

These are used to assess acid reflux. A probe is inserted via the nose down the oesophagus and records pH. Regular falls in pH are associated with acid reflux.

Helicobacter pylori testing

Helicobacter pylori is an important factor in the pathogenesis of peptic ulcer and should be tested for in cases of dyspepsia, especially if the patient has peptic ulcers. Testing can be by:

- Histology.
- Urease testing of biopsies—campylobacter-like organism (CLO) test. Biopsies are placed in a small amount of medium containing urea. Helicobacter splits urea to form ammonia, which turns a pH indicator in the medium bright pink.

- Presence of antibodies in the blood (enzyme-linked immunosorbent assay).
- Breath (^{13}C urea) test—urea containing ^{13}C is fed to the patient and helicobacter splits it, creating $^{13}CO_2$, which is detected in exhaled breath.

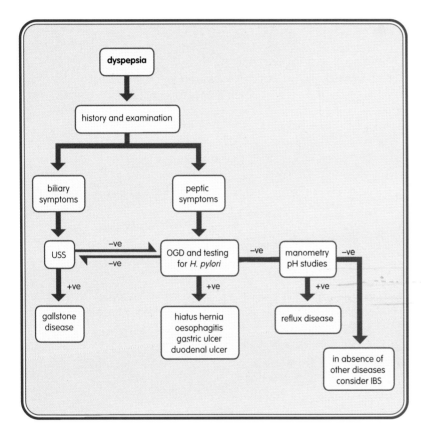

Fig. 2.1 Investigation and diagnosis of dyspepsia. (IBS, irritable bowel syndrome; OGD, oesophagogastroduodenoscopy; USS, ultrasound scan.)

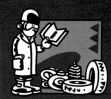

3. Vomiting, Haematemesis, and Melaena

Vomiting is a common consequence of many non-specific illnesses. If the vomitus contains blood the vomiting is termed haematemesis. The blood may be either fresh red blood or partly digested blood, which often has the appearance of 'coffee grounds'.

Melaena is the passage of altered blood rectally and is characterized by offensive smelling, black, tarry stool.

Both haematemesis and melaena represent bleeding from the upper gastrointestinal tract. Bleeding from the lower gastrointestinal tract is dealt with in Chapter 6

DIFFERENTIAL DIAGNOSIS OF VOMITING, HAEMATEMESIS, AND MELAENA

The differential diagnosis of vomiting includes:
- Mechanical obstruction (of oesophagus, stomach, small bowel, or large bowel).
- Obstruction of other smooth muscle tubes. (e.g. biliary ducts, ureter, fallopian tube, appendix).
- Irritation of nerves of peritoneum or mesentery (e.g. due to perforation of viscus, intra-abdominal sepsis, torted ovarian cyst, gastritis).
- Chemically induced (e.g. by drugs, alcohol).
- Central nervous system disorders (e.g. vestibulitis, motion sickness).

The differential diagnosis of haematemesis, and melaena includes:
- Peptic ulcer (duodenal or gastric ulcer).
- Gastric erosions.
- Oesophagitis.
- Mallory–Weiss tear.
- Oesophageal or gastric malignancy.
- Oesophageal varices.

HISTORY TO FOCUS ON THE DIFFERENTIAL DIAGNOSIS OF VOMITING, HAEMATEMESIS, AND MELAENA

Pain
Pain often precedes the vomiting and its location can help to diagnose the primary cause (see Chapter 1). Colicky abdominal pain is associated with obstruction of a viscus. Dyspepsia is associated with several causes of haematemesis (see above and Chapter 2).

Causes of obstruction of any tube are either:
- In the lumen
- In the wall
- Outside the wall

Timing of vomiting relative to food
Generally speaking the higher the obstruction the sooner the vomiting occurs after drinking (Fig. 3.1):
- Oesophageal obstruction—immediate vomiting.
- Gastric outlet obstruction—within 30 min.
- Small bowel obstruction—after several hours.
- Large bowel obstruction—vomiting may not occur until very late in the disease process.

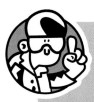

Common causes of small intestinal obstruction are:
- Irreducible hernias
- Adhesions

Features of vomiting			
Nature	Timing after eating	Associated symptoms	Site of problem
undigested food	immediately	dysphagia	oesophagus, gastric cardia
partially digested food	soon	epigastric pain	stomach, duodenum
bilious, partially digested food	few hours	abdominal distension, abdominal pain	small bowel
bilious, no food	any	dizziness	neurogenic, vestibular
haematemesis	any		oesophagus, stomach, duodenum

Fig. 3.1 Features of vomiting.

Content of the vomitus

The content of the vomitus gives some indication (in the case of obstruction) of the level involved:

- Food and acid—suggests gastric outflow obstruction due to either pyloric ulcer, duodenal ulcer, or carcinoma of the stomach.
- Bile—suggests obstruction distal to the sphincter of Oddi. It may also be seen with a gastritic-type picture when there is some reflux of bile into the stomach.
- Faeculent—indicates distal small bowel obstruction. The liquid is contaminated with bacterial flora, hence the faeculent nature.
- Fresh blood—indicates a recent fairly brisk bleed.
- 'Coffee grounds'—indicate a less recent or 'not so severe' bleed.

Symptoms of intestinal obstruction are:
- **Colicky abdominal pain**
- **Abdominal distension**
- **Vomiting**
- **Absolute constipation**

Nausea and loss of appetite

An acute loss of appetite is always important and should be investigated further.

Drug history

Many drugs have side effects of nausea and vomiting. This may be due to a central action or a direct irritant action on the stomach mucosa.

Some drugs are associated with upper gastrointestinal haemorrhage, for example:

- Non-steroidal anti-inflammatory drugs.
- Corticosteroids.

Chronic cigarette smoking and alcohol intake predispose to peptic ulceration, which is the commonest cause of haematemesis.

EXAMINATION OF PATIENTS WHO HAVE VOMITING, HAEMATEMESIS, AND MELAENA

General examination

Weight loss may indicate malignancy.

Longstanding gastric outflow problems due to benign disease can also lead to nutritional deficits.

Persistent vomiting results in dehydration, which may manifest as decreased skin turgor, tachycardia, hypotension, and low urine output.

Marked blood loss from haematemesis and melaena cause anaemia and cardiovascular collapse.

Abdominal examination

For the most part this is the same as for an acute abdomen (see Chapter 1 and Part II), but several specific features may be associated with vomiting:

- Scars of previous abdominal operations.
- Large palpable gastric tumours.
- In neonates the mass of a pyloric stenosis may be palpable as a small mass in the epigastrium on test feeding.

- An irreducible tender hernia may be the cause of intestinal obstruction.

Succussion splash
This is due to chronic gastric outflow obstruction and is produced because the distended stomach contains fluid and gas.

INVESTIGATION OF PATIENTS WHO HAVE VOMITING, HAEMATEMESIS, AND MELAENA

An algorithm for the investigation and diagnosis of vomiting, haematemesis, and melaena is given in Fig. 3.2.

Blood tests
Full blood count
This may show:
- Anaemia—associated with haematemesis or melaena or due to chronic blood loss.
- Increased white cell count—in infection.
- Increased haematocrit—in dehydration due to persistent vomiting.

Urea and electrolytes
Measurement of urea and electrolytes including chloride may show:
- Increased urea and creatinine levels—seen in dehydration.
- Increased urea but normal creatinine—seen in upper gastrointestinal haemorrhage.
- Low chloride—in gastric outflow obstruction due to loss of hydrochloric acid in the vomitus.

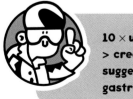

10 × urea (mmol/L) > creatinine (mmol/L) suggests an upper gastrointestinal bleed.

Blood gases
Loss of hydrochloric acid in gastric outflow obstruction leads to an alkalosis. This in turn can lead to a hypokalaemia as the kidneys try to preserve hydrogen ions (H^+) at the expense of potassium ions (K^+).

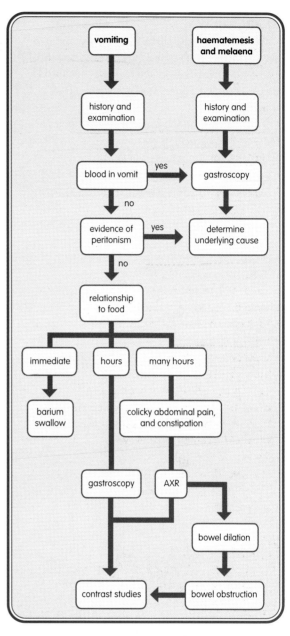

Fig. 3.2 Investigation and diagnosis of vomiting, haematemesis and melaena. (AXR, abdominal radiography.)

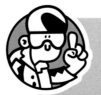

Using a urine dipstick to test vomit for blood is a waste of time. Vomitus invariably contains sufficient traces of haemoglobin to cause a positive reaction.

15

Radiography
Abdominal radiography
Dilated small or large bowel may be seen on plain abdominal radiography and the level of obstruction can be estimated. Some distinguishing features include:

- Small bowel is arranged more centrally and has bands that traverse its entire diameter (the plicae circulares or valvulae coniventes).
- Large bowel lies more peripherally and has bands (haustra) that do not extend across its diameter.
- Both large and small bowel may be distended if there is large bowel obstruction with an incompetent ileocaecal valve.
- A caecum of more than 10 cm in diameter is at risk of perforation.

Other features may also show up on a plain abdominal radiograph such as:

- Ureteric stone—over 90% are visible on plain film.
- Gallstone—less than 10% are visible on plain film.

Chest radiography
An erect chest radiograph can show free gas under the diaphragm indicating a perforated viscus that may be causing peritonitis

Contrast studies
Barium swallow can be used to investigate vomiting due to oesophageal or gastric pathology. In suspected small bowel obstruction, a barium follow-through can be performed to assess the level of obstruction. An unprepared barium enema can show obstructing lesions in the colon.

Oesophagogastroduodenoscopy
This is used to diagnose causes of haematemesis and melaena including:

- Oesophagitis.
- Gastritis.
- Gastric ulcer.
- Duodenal ulcer.
- Gastric and oesophageal cancer.

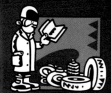

4. Change in Bowel Habit

Normal bowel habit is a very variable phenomenon. It can range from three to four times a day to just once a week. The frequency and consistency of stool is not the most important finding, but the change in habit is.

DIFFERENTIAL DIAGNOSIS OF A CHANGE IN BOWEL HABIT

The differential diagnoses are:
- Colonic carcinoma.
- Ulcerative colitis.
- Crohn's disease.
- Diverticular disease.
- Benign colonic polyps.
- Infective causes (including parasitic infection).
- Anal carcinoma.
- Endocrine disorders.

HISTORY TO FOCUS ON THE DIFFERENTIAL DIAGNOSIS OF A CHANGE IN BOWEL HABIT

Constipation or diarrhoea
Ask the patient how the bowel habit has changed. Worsening diarrhoea may be associated with inflammatory bowel disease, infective colitis, villous adenoma and colonic carcinoma.

The patient may complain of increasing difficulty in opening the bowels suggestive of:
- Stenosing carcinoma of the colon and especially rectum.
- Diverticular stricture
- Hypothyroidism.

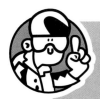

Left-sided colonic tumours can cause constipation or diarrhoea.

Associated symptoms
Rectal blood or mucus
Blood may be passed in the stool with or without mucus (see Chapter 6):
- Fresh blood—usually due to anorectal disease, either a carcinoma, polyp, or perianal disease.
- Dark blood (partly altered blood)—usually from the sigmoid colon or above.
- Mixed with stool—usually above the sigmoid colon (stool is softer and has time to mix with the blood).
- Blood and mucus—inflammatory bowel disease or colorectal carcinoma.
- Mucus but no blood—typically seen in irritable bowel syndrome.

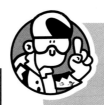

Villous adenomas cause diarrhoea as a result of excess mucus production and may cause hypokalaemia.

Pain
The patient may complain of abdominal pain associated with the change in bowel habit. This may be:
- Colicky central abdominal pain (small bowel colic). If associated with diarrhoea the cause may be infective diarrhoea or Crohn's disease, but may be a feature of small bowel obstruction due to a caecal cancer.
- Colicky lower abdominal pain is usually associated with colonic pathology. If associated with absolute constipation it can be a sign of complete bowel obstruction. Localized sharp pain in the left iliac fossa may be due to diverticulitis.

Weight loss
Weight loss may be seen with:
- Inflammatory bowel disease, especially Crohn's disease.
- Carcinoma of the bowel.

Tenesmus
This describes the sensation of incomplete emptying of the rectum. It is usually associated with a rectal mass lesion, either carcinoma or a large polyp, but may also be seen in inflammatory bowel disease affecting the rectum.

Abdominal distension
This may be due to either obstruction of the bowel or ascites (see Chapter 5). Patients who have irritable bowel also describe bloating of the abdomen usually following meals which may be associated with colicky abdominal pain

Family history
Certain conditions may be hereditary, for example:
- Familial polyposis coli—autosomal dominant inheritance.
- Carcinoma of the bowel—increased risk if a relative under 50 years of age has carcinoma of the bowel.
- Inflammatory bowel disease—associated with certain major histocompatibility antigens (e.g. HLA-B27).

Social history
Foreign travel is common these days and acquired infective causes should be sought. Common infections include:
- Giardiasis.
- Shigellosis.
- Salmonellosis.
- Campylobacter infection.

Less common infections are:
- Amoebic dysentery.
- Typhoid.
- Cholera.

Drug history
Many drugs can cause constipation including:
- Opioid analgesics.
- Anticholinergics.
- Antidiarrhoeal medication.

Others drugs cause diarrhoea including:
- Laxatives.
- Antibiotics.

Antibiotics can also destroy the natural flora of the gut and so lead to pseudomembranous colitis.

EXAMINATION OF PATIENTS WHO HAVE A CHANGE IN BOWEL HABIT

General examination
Look for signs of:
- Anaemia—due to blood loss from the gastrointestinal tract from a polyp or malignancy. Anaemia may also result from malabsorption of vitamin B_{12} due to terminal ileal disease in Crohn's disease.
- Weight loss.
- Jaundice—due to metastases from carcinoma of the bowel
- Lymphadenopathy—especially Virchow's node in the left supraclavicular fossa associated with intra-abdominal malignancy.
- Clubbing—may be seen in inflammatory bowel disease.
- Skin changes—both pyoderma gangrenosum and erythema nodosum are associated with inflammatory bowel disease.

Mouth
Inspection of the mouth may reveal:
- Pigmentation of buccal mucosa—associated with Peutz–Jeghers syndrome.
- Aphthous ulcers—seen in Crohn's disease.

Abdominal examination
This is carried out as for the acute abdomen (see p. 99) paying particular attention to the presence of:
- Masses—associated with colonic carcinoma, diverticular disease, or Crohn's disease.
- Tenderness—diverticulitis (see Chapter 1).

Rectal examination
This is essential for the patient who has a change of bowel habit. Many rectal tumours are low enough to be palpated.

INVESTIGATION OF PATIENTS WHO HAVE A CHANGE IN BOWEL HABIT

An algorithm for the investigation and diagnosis of patients who have a change in bowel habit is given in Fig. 4.1.

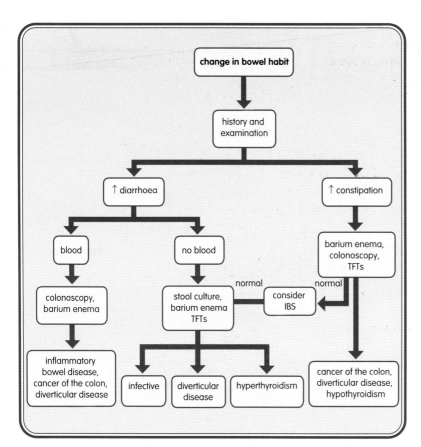

Fig. 4.1 Investigation and diagnosis of a change in bowel habit. (IBS, irritable bowel syndrome; TFTs, thyroid function tests.)

Blood tests
Full blood count
A hypochromic microcytic anaemia is associated with a chronic blood loss (e.g. due to carcinoma of the bowel). A macrocytic picture may be associated with malabsorption due to terminal ileal Crohn's disease.

White cell count
This can be increased in infective diarrhoea, but may also be increased in active inflammatory bowel disease.

Thyroid function tests
The thyrotoxic patient may have diarrhoea, whereas the myxoedematous patient may be constipated.

C-reactive protein and erythrocyte sedimentation rate
These markers of acute inflammation are fairly non-specific, but are markedly increased in inflammatory bowel disease.

Carcinoembryonic antigen
This tumour marker may be increased in carcinoma of the colon.

Stool culture and microscopy
Cultures should be sent to diagnose bacterial causes of diarrhoea.

Microscopy should be performed for parasitic infections.

Tests for *Clostridium difficile* toxin should be performed if pseudomembranous colitis is suspected.

Endoscopy
Rigid sigmoidoscopy
Sigmoidoscopy allows visualization of the rectum and lower sigmoid. Any neoplastic lesions or inflammatory changes in this area can be seen and biopsied.

Flexible sigmoidoscopy and colonoscopy
This allows visualization of a greater extent of the colon and biopsies can be taken or polyps removed.

19

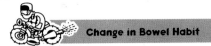

Radiography
Double contrast barium enema
This gives good imaging of the colonic mucosa. It may be useful for visualizing bowel:

- Proximal to a stricture through which a colonoscope cannot pass.
- If colonoscopy is not possible because the colon is tortuous or there is severe diverticulosis.

5. Abdominal Mass and Distension

It is rare for a patient to present with an abdominal mass as a primary symptom. Usually it is a discovery made after presentation with other symptoms. Abdominal swelling, however, is often noticed by the patient when clothes no longer fit.

DIFFERENTIAL DIAGNOSIS OF ABDOMINAL MASS OR DISTENSION

The differential diagnosis of abdominal masses is given in Fig. 5.1.

The classical causes of abdominal distension are the five Fs:

- Fat.
- Flatus.
- Faeces.
- Fluid.
- Foetus.

To these must be added the more specific diagnoses:

- Tumour.
- Inflammatory mass.
- Aneurysm.
- Hernia.
- Organomegaly (including bladder).

HISTORY TO FOCUS ON THE DIFFERENTIAL DIAGNOSIS OF ABDOMINAL MASS OR DISTENSION

Timing

Take a careful history of how the swelling has developed:

- A rapid onset of generalized swelling is associated with a bowel obstruction.
- A rapid onset of painful lower abdominal swelling can occur if there is acute retention of urine.
- Other causes of swelling usually take much longer to increase in size or for the patient to become aware of it.

Associated symptoms

The clinician should be alerted to the possibility of bowel obstruction when a patient presents with the following symptoms, especially in the presence of colicky abdominal pain:

- Nausea.
- Vomiting.
- Absolute constipation (passing neither faeces nor flatus).

The classical history of ascites is a long history of increasing abdominal distension without much pain,

Differential diagnosis of abdominal masses	
Location	Differential diagnosis
epigastric	hepatomegaly gastric tumour pancreatic tumour transverse colon tumour pancreatic pseudocyst
right hypochondrium	distended gall bladder cancer of the hepatic flexure of the colon hepatomegaly
left hypochondrium	splenomegaly cancer of the descending colon pancreatic pseudocyst
right iliac fossa	distended caecum caecal tumour appendix mass Crohn's disease ovarian mass
left iliac fossa	sigmoid colon tumour diverticular abscess or mass ovarian mass constipation
flank	renal tumour polycystic kidney
suprapubic	distended bladder uterus—fibroids, uterine cancer, pregnancy! ovarian mass

Fig. 5.1 Differential diagnosis of abdominal masses.

but associated with swelling of the legs and shortness of breath. The shortness of breath is due to splinting of the diaphragm with increasing pressure in the abdomen, but may also be associated with a pleural effusion, which is seen in about 60% of patients who have ascites.

Pain

If pain is associated with the swelling, its character and site can give some clue about the nature of the swelling:

- Back pain is associated with retroperitoneal structures such as the pancreas and aorta. Pancreatic malignancy can present as an unrelenting back pain due to direct invasion by the tumour.
- Aortic aneurysms can present with different types of pain. There is the dull pain in the back associated with direct pressure of the aneurysm. The pain may become more intense as the aorta stretches rapidly. There is also the severe pain of dissection or rupture.
- Hernias rarely cause severe pain except when they become strangulated. They may also present with obstruction.
- Symptoms of rapidly expanding organs such as the liver and spleen can cause abdominal pain due to distension of their relatively inelastic capsules.

Identify symptoms of malignancy

Any of the following symptoms may be due to underlying malignancy:

- Unexplained weight loss.
- Anorexia.
- Change in bowel habit.
- Night sweats.

Careful direct questioning about these symptoms is required.

Malignancy may be the underlying cause of many of the differential diagnoses including:

- Ascites—due to peritoneal spread of tumour.
- Hernia—due to straining to pass a stool by a patient who has carcinoma of the rectum.
- Hepatomegaly—due to metastatic disease.
- Bowel obstruction—due to direct mechanical obstruction by tumour.

Drug history

Some drug therapies can cause abdominal swelling:

- Opioid analgesics can cause severe constipation.
- Many psychotropic drugs can cause bowel inactivity leading to pseudo-obstruction of the bowel.

- α-Blockers (α-adrenoceptor antagonists) can cause urinary retention leading to an enlarged bladder.
- Corticosteroid therapy results in deposition of body fat in a central distribution and can lead to increased abdominal fat layers.

EXAMINATION OF PATIENTS WHO HAVE ABDOMINAL MASS OR DISTENSION

General examination

The clinician should observe general signs such as anaemia, weight loss and lymphadenopathy, which may indicate underlying malignancy. Signs of liver failure suggesting that the swelling is due to ascites include:

- Palmar erythema.
- Jaundice.
- Spider naevi (more than five on the body).
- Liver flap.

Cardiovascular examination

Absent peripheral pulses and poor circulation indicate atherosclerotic disease and an increased risk of aneurysmal disease. Peripheral oedema may be associated with ascites of any cause, but may also be a sign of congestive cardiac failure with hepatomegaly, and ascites.

Respiratory examination

Watching the patient breathe may reveal some signs of diaphragmatic splinting and auscultation may reveal small effusions associated with ascites.

Abdominal examination

Inspection will indicate whether abdominal swelling is generalized such as ascites or just a localized swelling. Redness or oedema of skin over the swelling can indicate local inflammation. Distended abdominal wall veins are seen in patients who have liver disease and ascites.

Palpation

The clinician is able to tell on palpation whether the swelling is generalized and whether there is an underlying local cause. The position of any mass and a knowledge of abdominal anatomy is crucial to aiding differential diagnosis (see Fig. 5.1)

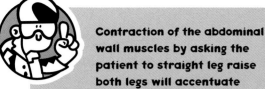

Contraction of the abdominal wall muscles by asking the patient to straight leg raise both legs will accentuate abdominal wall masses and hernias. Deep masses will be impalpable with the abdominal muscles contracted.

Hepatomegaly and splenomegaly can extend into the right iliac fossa. Start in the right iliac fossa when attempting to identify these masses.

Percussion

Distended bowel associated with obstruction is hyperresonant. Shifting dullness is pathognomonic of ascites.

Auscultation

High-pitched tinkling bowel sounds are associated with bowel obstruction. Absent bowel sounds can indicate an ileus or pseudo-obstruction.

INVESTIGATION OF PATIENTS WHO HAVE ABDOMINAL MASS OR DISTENSION

An algorithm for the investigation and diagnosis of abdominal swelling is given in Fig. 5.2.

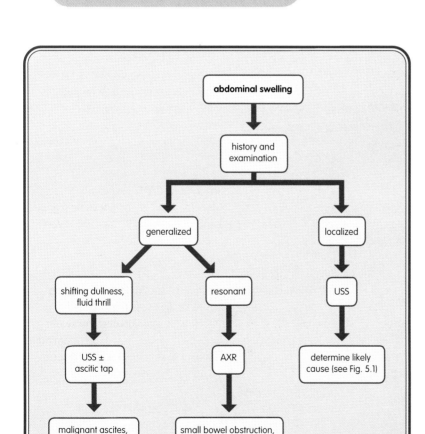

Fig. 5.2 Investigation and diagnosis of an abdominal swelling. (AXR, abdominal radiography; USS, ultrasound scan.)

Blood tests
Full blood count
An increased white cell count may be associated with bowel obstruction as well as inflammatory masses.

Liver function tests
These may show liver dysfunction. A low albumin is a marker of poor liver synthetic function and may also cause ascites.

Tumour markers
These include:
- Carcinoembryonic antigen (CEA)—a marker for colonic carcinoma.
- CA125—a marker for ovarian carcinoma.
- β-Human chorionic gonadotrophin (BHCG) —a marker for teratoma.
- α-Fetoprotein (AFP)—a marker for primary hepatoma and teratoma.

Radiography
Abdominal radiography
Distended loops of bowel filled with gas or fluid are indicative of obstruction or pseudo-obstruction. Distended loops of small bowel indicate small bowel obstruction whereas colonic or pseudo-obstruction is indicated if there is colonic dilatation with or without small bowel dilatation. A 'ground glass' appearance suggests the presence of ascites.

Ultrasonography
This can reveal:
- Ascites.
- Abnormally enlarged organs.
- Malignant masses.
- Large cysts in ovaries or kidneys.
- Abscesses.
- Inflammatory masses.

Computed tomography
This may show the same pathology as ultrasonography, but is more useful in showing retroperitoneal structures.

Special investigations
Ascitic tap
This is used to:
- Assess the protein content of the ascites to determine its aetiology (i.e. whether it is a transudate or an exudate).
- Look for the presence of malignant cells.

Biopsy
A fine-needle aspiration cytology, core biopsy, or ultrasound-guided biopsy of a mass or palpable lymphadenopathy can provide a histological diagnosis.

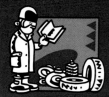

6. Rectal Bleeding

This chapter is concerned with the causes of fresh rectal bleeding. Rectal bleeding can be a source of great embarrassment for patients and they may suffer with the problem for a long time before presenting to a clinician. A sudden onset of a large volume of rectal bleeding may be a reason for an acute surgical admission.

- Diverticular disease.
- Ischaemic colitis.

Patients who have a colonic carcinoma may also have haemorrhoids. Do not assume rectal bleeding is due to the presence of haemorrhoids.

DIFFERENTIAL DIAGNOSIS OF RECTAL BLEEDING

The differential diagnoses of rectal bleeding (Fig. 6.1) are:
- Haemorrhoids.
- Fissure in ano.
- Inflammatory bowel disease.
- Rectal polyp or adenoma.
- Carcinoma of the colon, rectum, or anus.
- Angiodysplasia of the colon.

HISTORY TO FOCUS ON THE DIFFERENTIAL DIAGNOSIS OF RECTAL BLEEDING

Age
Haemorrhoids and fissure in ano are prevalent at every age. Diverticular disease and cancer are rare in people under 40 years of age.

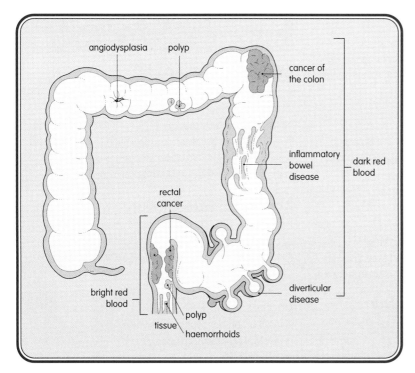

Fig. 6.1 Causes of rectal bleeding.

Character of the bleeding

Bright red blood is usually indicative of anorectal pathology. Dark altered blood is associated with colonic pathology and occasionally it is due to a brisk bleed from an upper gastrointestinal source.

Upper gastrointestinal bleeding is usually darker in nature (i.e. melaena; see Chapter 3).

Relationship of bleeding to stool

Mixed with stool

Blood mixed with the stool is indicative of a bleeding source high up in the colon. The softer stool and time taken to evacuate stool from here means that the blood and stool can mix. It is unusual for this to happen as a result of bleeding from a site below the descending colon.

On surface of the stool

Blood on the surface of the stool is usually from the sigmoid colon or lower. Isolated streaks of blood on the stool and associated with severe pain on defecation is associated with fissure in ano.

Blood separate from stool

Blood that is separate from stool is usually produced after defaecation and is associated with anorectal conditions such as haemorrhoids. The patient will often describe dripping of blood into the toilet after defaecation.

Blood on the toilet paper

This is usually associated with anorectal conditions such as haemorrhoids and fissures where the bleeding is not as brisk and a small bloody residue is left on the anal skin.

Mucus

A discharge of mucus may accompany the bleeding if it is due to ulcerative colitis or Crohn's disease of the rectum or if the bleeding is due to an adenoma.

Associated symptoms

Pain

Anorectal pain is not usually a major feature of haemorrhoids or carcinoma of the colon (see Chapter 7).

Severe pain on defaecation may be associated with an anal fissure.

Abdominal pain can be associated with inflammatory bowel disease or ischaemic colitis.

Colicky abdominal pain is a feature of an impending obstruction from a carcinoma of the colon (see Chapter 1).

Angiodysplasia of the colon or diverticular disease may cause sudden brisk painless bleeding with clots.

Change in bowel habit

Change in bowel habit is discussed in Chapter 4.

Tenesmus

Tenesmus is a feeling of incomplete evacuation. It is usually caused by a space-occupying lesion of the rectum, but may also be associated with acute inflammatory conditions of the rectum.

Weight loss

In the elderly, this suggests malignancy, but in the younger patient inflammatory bowel disease such as Crohn's disease or ulcerative colitis is more likely.

Family history

Some patients have several first degree relatives who have had carcinoma of the bowel and their risk of developing bowel cancer may be as high as 1 in 2 based on 'cancer family' genetic screening.

Familial polyposis coli, in which patients have more than 100 polyps in the colon, is an autosomal dominant condition and is associated with an almost 100% risk of developing bowel cancer.

EXAMINATION OF PATIENTS WHO HAVE RECTAL BLEEDING

General examination

A general examination of the patient is carried out, looking in particular for clinical signs of anaemia associated with chronic blood loss. If the patient has been admitted as an acute admission to hospital and has marked rectal bleeding, his or her pulse, blood pressure, and urine output must be monitored.

Abdominal examination

This is often normal, but there may be a palpable mass due to a colonic tumour or an inflammatory mass due to Crohn's disease, or tenderness associated with ischaemic colitis.

Anal inspection

Inspection of the anus may reveal:
- Prolapsed haemorrhoids.
- Anal fissure.

- Anal tumours.
- Prolapsing low rectal tumour.
- Skin tags—which may be associated with fissures and fistulae.
- Perianal sepsis—which may be associated with Crohn's disease.

Digital rectal examination

Insertion of a finger into the rectum can reveal many conditions:

- A fissure may be palpable as an exquisitely tender induration.
- The sphincter tone is usually high in patients who have a fissure, and examination may not be possible.
- Low rectal tumours are palpable up to 7 cm.

Proctoscopy and sigmoidoscopy

The proctoscope is used to look for anorectal problems and can be particularly useful for visualizing haemorrhoids, which are impalpable.

The sigmoidoscope is used to provide a view of the rectum and the lower sigmoid colon. Lesions can be directly inspected and biopsied.

INVESTIGATION OF PATIENTS WHO HAVE RECTAL BLEEDING

An algorithm for the investigation and diagnosis of rectal bleeding is given in Fig. 6.2.

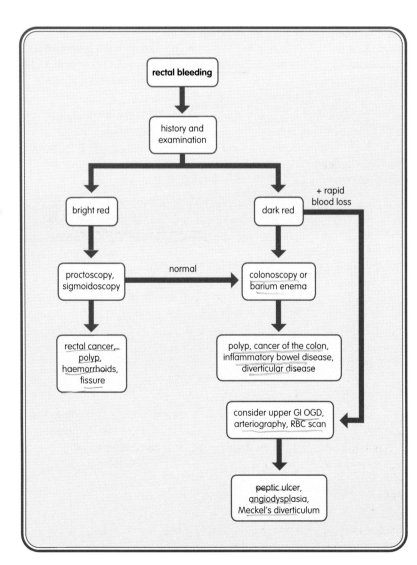

Fig. 6.2 Investigation and diagnosis of rectal bleeding. (GI, gastrointestinal; OGD, oesophagogastroduodenoscopy; RBC, red blood cell.)

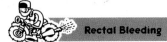
Blood tests
Full blood count
This provides an assessment of the degree of blood loss. Chronic blood loss will be reflected as a hypochromic microcytic anaemia.

Haemorrhoids do not bleed sufficiently to cause anaemia.

Carcinoembryonic antigen
This tumour marker can be increased in colonic carcinoma (see Chapter 5).

Barium enema and colonoscopy
A flexible colonoscopic investigation has advantages over barium enema because it is the only method for visualizing areas of angiodysplasia and small polyps.

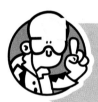

Lesions below the dentate line should not be biopsied without anaesthesia.

Further investigations
Gastroscopy
This is not usually a first-line investigation for rectal bleeding, but if there has been marked loss of dark blood a bleeding peptic ulcer may be the cause.

Labelled red cell scan
This is mainly used for diagnosing bleeding from a Meckel's diverticulum or if other tests are normal.

Angiography
This is a specialized investigation to identify the bleeding source if there is rapid bleeding and surgical intervention may be required. A radio-opaque contrast is selectively injected into each mesenteric artery in turn and screening is used to show the site of blood loss into the gut. The patient has to be bleeding at 1–1.5 mL/min for the test to be helpful.

The usual causes of rapid blood loss from the colon are bleeding from a diverticulum or angiodysplasia.

7. Anorectal Pain

Anorectal pain, like rectal bleeding, is a cause of embarrassment for many patients and it may be suffered for some time before the patient seeks professional help.

DIFFERENTIAL DIAGNOSIS OF ANORECTAL PAIN

The differential diagnoses of anorectal pain are:
- Fissure in ano.
- Perianal haematoma.
- Thrombosed haemorrhoids.
- Fistula in ano.
- Perianal abscess.
- Local irritation (pruritus ani).
- Carcinoma of the rectum or anus.
- Coccydynia.
- Proctalgia fugax.
- Pilonidal abscess.

HISTORY TO FOCUS ON THE DIFFERENTIAL DIAGNOSIS OF ANORECTAL PAIN

Pain

A history of the nature of the pain should be taken as with all painful complaints, but particular attention should be paid to the timing of the anal pain (i.e. in relation to defecation).
- Severe anal pain at the time of defecation that eases off afterwards is often associated with an anal fissure.
- Sudden onset of pain and swelling after passing a bulky stool may indicate a perianal haematoma or prolapsed haemorrhoids.

Abscesses usually present with a gradual onset of throbbing pain that increases in intensity, but may be suddenly relieved if the contents discharge (see below).

The patient may indicate the site of the pain as external and describe the pain as 'soreness'. This is usually associated with local skin irritation.

Carcinoma of the rectum or anus does not usually present with anal pain, but if there is pain this often indicates invasion of the tumour into the anal sphincter. The pain is usually severe and persistent without any respite and no exacerbating factors.

A history of a fall onto the base of the spine in recent months followed by pain on opening the bowels may suggest a coccygeal injury.

The patient may describe a sharp shooting pain of sudden onset that is deep inside the anal canal and often occurs at night. There appears to be no relation to bowel habit and the pain disappears quickly. This is the typical presentation of proctalgia fugax (flitting anal pain).

Bleeding

Causes of rectal bleeding are dealt with in Chapter 6 and the history should be taken in the manner described.

Discharge

A history of any discharge or 'wetness' should be obtained. Patients often do not describe a discharge, but on direct questioning may describe staining of underwear or even some soiling. Nearly all of the diagnoses mentioned in this chapter can lead to some form of excess moisture in the perianal region and may also cause local irritation of the skin externally. Faecal soiling of the underwear raises the possibility of a fistula.

EXAMINATION OF PATIENTS WHO HAVE ANORECTAL PAIN

General examination of the patient should of course be carried out in all cases. Attention should be paid to:
- Signs of weight loss—should alert the clinician to malignancy or Crohn's disease.
- Anaemia—due to severe rectal bleeding
- Pyrexia and tachycardia—indicate a source of sepsis.

Inspection

Close inspection of the external anal skin may reveal excoriated inflamed skin.

Skin tags may be associated with fissure in ano and multiple skin tags can be associated with Crohn's disease.

An abscess may be visible as an obvious swelling in the perianal region with reddened overlying skin.

There may be a small perianal opening discharging pus or faecal material. The position of the opening should be noted because it will guide the clinician in looking for the internal communication of a fistula. Fistulae with anterior external openings open directly into the anal canal or rectum, whereas fistulae with external openings posterior to the midline usually open in the midline of the anal canal or rectum (Goodsall's rule, Fig. 7.1).

Thrombosed piles and perianal haematomas may be confused, but several differences will distinguish one from the other:

- Thrombosed piles are recognized as dark blue swellings protruding from the anal canal covered in oedematous dusky mucosa.
- Perianal haematomas are subcutaneous swellings on the anal verge and are covered in skin.
- Thrombosed piles are exquisitely tender to touch.
- Perianal haematomas, although causing quite marked pain to the patient are generally not tender to the touch.

If the piles have been prolapsed and thrombosed for some time they may be excoriated and ulcerated and may be confused with a protruding anorectal carcinoma.

Pilonidal abscesses usually lie in the natal cleft and there may be associated midline pits. In all cases of pilonidal abscess there is association with excess hair in the natal cleft.

Digital rectal examination

Once inspection of the external anus has been completed a gloved finger should be inserted. Occasionally digital rectal examination is not possible because of severe pain and in this case no further investigation should be performed without anaesthetic. Features to look for include:

- Sphincter tone—this should be judged and is usually high in patients who have anal fissure.
- Any irregularity in the anal canal—anal fissures are often palpable as small indurated or even 'sharp' lesions on the anal verge. The patient will tell you that touching this area is extremely painful.

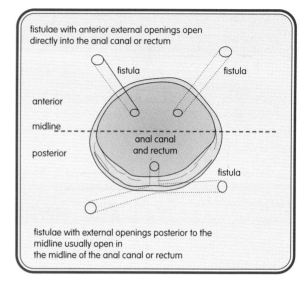

Fig. 7.1 Goodsall's rule.

- Any palpable masses—both size and position (related to clockface) should be recorded.
- Prostatic features in the male (see Chapter 17).
- Coccygeal pain—the coccyx is palpable posteriorly and backward pressure over this causes severe pain in coccydynia.

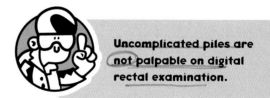

Uncomplicated piles are not palpable on digital rectal examination.

INVESTIGATION OF PATIENTS WHO HAVE ANORECTAL PAIN

An algorithm for the investigation and diagnosis of anorectal pain is given in Fig. 7.2.

Proctoscopy and sigmoidoscopy

The anal canal and rectum should be inspected directly and attention paid to any mucosal abnormality. An internal opening to a fistula may be seen if there is discharge of pus into the rectum. Any lesions above the dentate line (the limit of somatic sensation in the anal canal) may be biopsied.

If digital rectal examination is not tolerated, sigmoidoscopy and proctoscopy are not advisable without anaesthesia (i.e. examination under anaesthetic —EUA).

Special investigations
Anorectal physiology

Assessment of sphincter pressure and coordination can be made with anorectal manometry. This may detect high pressures associated with anal fissures or painful spasms due to sphincter instability.

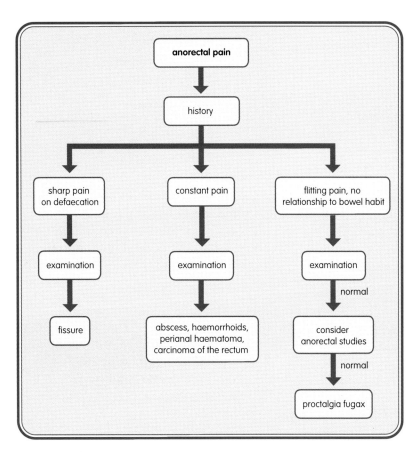

Fig. 7.2 Investigation and diagnosis of anorectal pain.

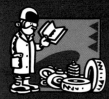

8. Jaundice

Jaundice describes the yellow discoloration of the skin associated with the deposition of bile pigments in the skin and sclera. It is clinically visible when serum bilirubin rises above 30 mmol/L.

Causes of jaundice can be split into prehepatic, hepatic, and posthepatic causes.

DIFFERENTIAL DIAGNOSIS OF JAUNDICE

The differential diagnoses of jaundice are:
- Prehepatic—haemolytic disorders, congenital hyperbilirubinaemias.
- Hepatic—viral hepatitis, alcoholic liver disease, cirrhosis, drug-induced, metastatic disease.
- Posthepatic—common bile duct stones, carcinoma of head of the pancreas, ampulla, or bile duct, biliary stricture (benign or malignant), external biliary compression (Mirrizzi's syndrome—i.e. gallstone impacted in the neck of the gall bladder, but compressing bile duct), enlarged nodes in the porta hepatis.

HISTORY TO FOCUS ON THE DIFFERENTIAL DIAGNOSIS OF JAUNDICE

Presentation of jaundice
The way the jaundice presents can be of value:
- Jaundice associated with a common bile duct stone is usually quite rapid in onset and painful.
- A past history of self-limiting transient episodes of jaundice suggests passage of smaller stones.
- Infectious hepatitis is usually preceded by a flu-like illness. The jaundice is usually gradual in onset and progressive.
- Carcinoma of the pancreas usually has an insidious onset of jaundice, but is progressive.

Urine and stool change
The change in urine colour to dark brown and the stool to pale off-white is classically associated with obstructive jaundice, but may not represent true posthepatic jaundice because 'medical' causes can cause compression of the intrahepatic bile ducts.

Pain
Any pain associated with the jaundice should be explored and noted:
- Intermittent severe pain is associated with biliary colic and common bile duct stones.
- A dull ache in the right upper quadrant can be associated with viral hepatitis and cholestatic jaundice of any cause that gives rise to oedema and swelling of the liver, stretching the liver capsule.
- Carcinoma of the pancreas can either present painlessly or if there is local invasion by the tumour it may cause severe relentless back pain.
- Haemolytic jaundice is painless.

Social history
The social history can give many clues when trying to establish 'non-surgical' causes of jaundice:
- History of contact with known hepatitis carriers, blood transfusion, history of intravenous drug abuse, and sexual liaisons with new partners (especially homosexual males) are all risk factors for viral hepatitis B and C.
- Foreign travel to the Far East and Asia may warn of contact with hepatitis A.
- Alcohol ingestion should also be noted to establish the risk of alcoholic liver disease.

Drug history
Recent medications should be recorded. Many drugs can cause cholestatic jaundice even after one dose (e.g. chlorpromazine).

Associated symptoms
Lethargy and general malaise along with a flu-like illness may be associated with hepatitis.

Haemolytic disorders also produce malaise and lethargy, but because of the anaemia also cause breathlessness and often weight loss.

The presence of rigors and high fevers should alert the clinician to the possibility of cholangitis.

Pruritus due to bile salts is a feature of posthepatic jaundice.

EXAMINATION OF PATIENTS WHO HAVE JAUNDICE

General examination

The clinician should look for evidence of recent weight loss. A careful search should also be made for stigmata of chronic liver disease (see Chapter 30, Fig. 30.2). Other physical signs are pyrexia, lymphadenopathy, and anaemia.

Abdominal examination

Inspection of the abdomen may reveal further evidence of liver disease:

- A caput medusae (distended veins around the umbilicus)—indicative of portal hypertension associated with chronic liver disease.
- Distension—due to gross ascites.

The size and texture of the liver should be noted:

- A large tender smooth liver is a feature of hepatitis.
- An enlarged irregular liver may indicate the presence of multiple metastases.

Other masses associated with jaundice may be:

- A palpable gall bladder below the liver. The presence of a palpable gall bladder is usually indicative that the jaundice is not due to stone disease and in many cases points towards biliary or pancreatic malignancy (Courvoisier's law, see Chapter 30, Fig. 30.7).
- Large pancreatic tumours.
- Gastric malignancies, which can cause lymphadenopathy around the porta hepatis giving rise to bile duct compression.
- Other abdominal primary malignancies leading to liver metastases.

Courvoisier's law—if in the presence of jaundice the gall bladder is palpable, then the jaundice is not usually due to gallstones.

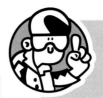

Murphy's sign—pressure in the right hypochondrium below the costal margin causes the patient to stop inspiration as the inflamed gall bladder impinges on the examiner's fingers. This is only positive in the absence of this sign in the left hypochondrium. It is a sign of cholecystitis.

Ascites may be present due to hypoproteinaemia associated with liver disease or an intra-abdominal malignancy including malignancy of the pancreas, stomach, colon, or ovary.

Abdominal examination should include a rectal examination. Pale stool may be seen or even a rectal tumour that has given rise to liver metastases.

INVESTIGATION OF PATIENTS WHO HAVE JAUNDICE

An algorithm for the investigation and diagnosis of jaundice is given in Fig. 8.1.

① Blood tests
Full blood count
This may show:

- Anaemia associated with haemolysis—if haemolysis is suspected a reticulocyte count should also be performed.
- An increased white cell count associated with sepsis. *+ cholecystitis*

② Liver function tests
These can give some indication to the cause of jaundice as well as some idea of the severity of disease:

- Alkaline phosphatase is a ductal enzyme and is increased in obstructive causes of jaundice.
- Alanine transaminase (ALT) and aspartate transaminase (AST) are hepatocellular enzymes, which are increased in hepatocellular dysfunction.

The results of liver function tests should never be interpreted in isolation because severe obstructive jaundice can cause hepatocellular failure.

· P·T + serum Albumin
+ · U+E's + Creat
· glucose · EBV, CMV, Hep·A, B, C

Amylase

Acute pancreatitis may be a sequel to obstructive jaundice due to a stone at the lower end of the common bile duct, but chronic pancreatitis may be the cause of bile duct obstruction.

Hepatitis serology

This should be checked if there is any possibility of past or present hepatitis infection.

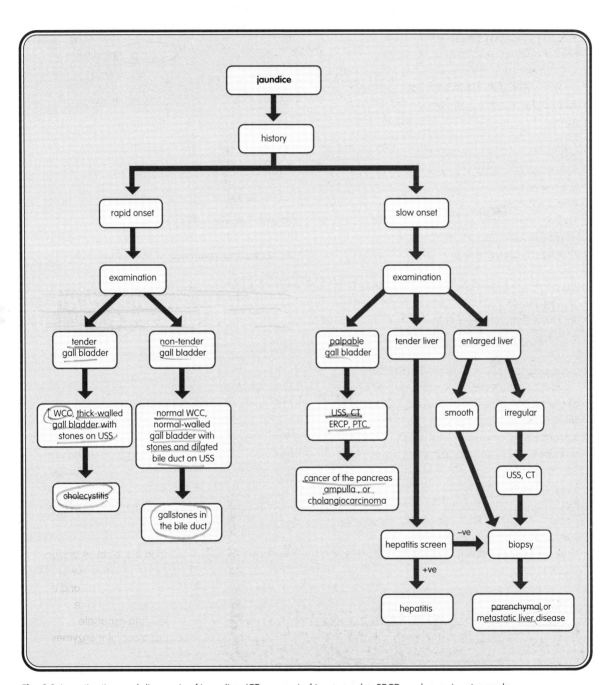

Fig. 8.1 Investigation and diagnosis of jaundice. (CT, computed tomography; ERCP, endoscopic retrograde cholangiopancreatography; PTC, percutaneous transhepatic cholangiography; USS, ultrasound scan; WCC, white cell count.)

35

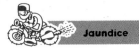

Urinalysis

The presence of bilirubin in the urine can be tested with a simple ward dipstick test. The presence of bilirubin in the urine demonstrates the presence of conjugated bilirubin, which is water-soluble. This indicates cholestasis or inability to excrete bilirubin due to:

- Hepatocellular dysfunction (intrahepatic cholestasis).
- Duct obstruction (extrahepatic cholestasis).

Jaundice without bilirubin in the urine is seen with:
- Haemolytic jaundice.
- The more common hyperbilirubinaemias such as Gilbert syndrome and Crigler–Najjar syndrome.

Ultrasonography

This is a very useful tool in the investigation of jaundice. It can demonstrate:

- Dilated biliary ducts (intra- and extrahepatic) associated with biliary obstruction.
- Common bile duct stones.
- Architectural disturbance of the liver itself in association with liver parenchymal disease.
- Metastases.
- Pancreatic swelling or masses.

Computed tomography

Plain or contrast-enhanced computed tomography (CT) may be performed. Computed tomography is better than ultrasound for imaging the pancreas and contrast-enhanced CT can provide good visualization of metastases. Computed tomography may also demonstrate other intra-abdominal malignancies.

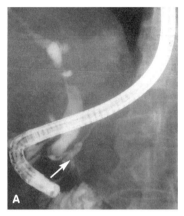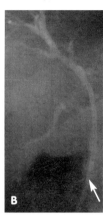

Fig. 8.2 **(A)** Endoscopic retrograde pancreatogram showing a stricture in the common bile duct (arrow) with **(B)** subsequent placement of a stent (arrow) across the stricture.

Cholangiography

This can be performed either by endoscopy (endoscopic retrograde cholangiopancreatography—ERCP) or by direct puncture of the intrahepatic ducts (percutaneous transhepatic cholangiography). Either of these methods can be used to demonstrate the presence of stones or tumour. In the case of ERCP a sphincterotomy can also be performed to remove stones or a stent can be inserted (Fig. 8.2) if there is a tumour.

Liver biopsy

When no extrahepatic cause for jaundice is found (i.e. there is no duct dilatation and no evidence of haemolysis) a liver biopsy may indicate the cause of liver dysfunction or provide histological proof of metastatic disease.

9. Dysphagia

Dysphagia is defined as difficulty in swallowing and may be associated with odynophagia, which is painful swallowing.

DIFFERENTIAL DIAGNOSIS OF DYSPHAGIA

The differential diagnosis of dysphagia is given in Fig. 9.1.

HISTORY TO FOCUS ON THE DIFFERENTIAL DIAGNOSIS OF DYSPHAGIA

Degree of dysphagia
The patient may have dysphagia only to solid foods such as meat and potatoes or may only be able to swallow liquids. Inability to swallow any fluid including saliva is a medical emergency and the patient requires immediate admission to hospital and investigation.

To ascertain the severity of dysphagia ask about the ease of swallowing the following foods—dysphagia is progressively worse as you move down the list:

- Meat
- Fish
- Mashed potatoes or vegetables
- Minced meat
- Liquids only

Onset
The onset and progression of dysphagia varies with the diagnosis:
- A sudden onset of dysphagia at the time of eating is suggestive of a bolus obstruction.
- A progressive dysphagia is commonly associated with malignancy.

Associated symptoms
Any associated symptoms should be elicited by direct questioning if necessary and may include:
- Dyspepsia—a long history of dyspepsia, reflux and progressive dysphagia is suggestive of benign stricture due to oesophageal reflux.
- Weight loss—may be associated with malignancy, but may just reflect the inability of the patient to ingest enough calories to maintain their normal weight due to severity of the dysphagia.
- Nocturnal cough—aspiration of the contents of a pharyngeal pouch or a dilated oesophagus may trickle down the trachea on lying flat at night, causing a coughing reflex.
- Haematemesis—this may arise from either a bleeding lesion in the oesophagus or may be related to a peptic ulcer (which may be associated with hyperacidity that also causes a stricture of the oesophagus).

Differential diagnosis of dysphagia	
Location	**Possible diagnoses**
in the lumen	foreign body
in the wall	inflammatory stricture caustic stricture achalasia tumour of oesophagus or gastric cardia pharyngeal pouch Plummer–Vinson syndrome diffuse oesophageal spasm scleroderma oesophageal web
outside the wall	retrosternal goitre enlarged left atrium bronchial carcinoma
general	bulbar palsy myaesthenia gravis hysteria

Fig. 9.1 Differential diagnosis of dysphagia.

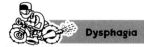

5 • Fatigue—may be due to anaemia, which may be secondary to upper gastrointestinal haemorrhage or chronic blood loss. Anaemia is also classically associated with Plummer–Vinson syndrome where it is linked to the presence of an oesophageal web.

6 • Breathlessness—this may be due to anaemia, but may also be associated with a bronchial carcinoma causing dysphagia or recurrent aspiration pneumonia.

7 • Other neurological symptoms—diseases such as polio, myasthenia gravis, bulbar palsy, and syringomyelia may lead to oesophageal motility problems and so questions about altered sensation and power (especially in the upper limbs) may be relevant.

EXAMINATION OF PATIENTS WHO HAVE DYSPHAGIA

Anaemia is very non-specific, but it is usually due to chronic blood loss from oesophageal carcinoma or gastric carcinoma or reflux oesophagitis.

Examination of the hands may reveal:
• Clubbing of the fingers—associated with a bronchial carcinoma.
• Waxy and tight fingers consistent with scleroderma or Raynaud's phenomenon—as part of CREST syndrome (Calcinosis, Raynaud's, (O)Esophageal motility disorders, Scleroderma, Telangiectasia).

Palpation of the neck may reveal lymphadenopathy in the supraclavicular fossa (Virchow's node) associated with a gastric or intrathoracic malignancy.

The thyroid can also be palpated to assess goitre (but enlargement of the thyroid causing dysphagia is usually retrosternal).

Respiratory examination including auscultation may reveal an underlying bronchial carcinoma or chest infection. A monophonic wheeze or pulmonary collapse may be diagnosed clinically.

INVESTIGATION OF PATIENTS WHO HAVE DYSPHAGIA

An algorithm for the investigation and diagnosis of dysphagia is given in Fig. 9.2.

Radiography
Chest radiography
This is a simple non-invasive investigation that may reveal:
• Primary lung carcinoma.
• Mediastinal mass.
• A large retrosternal goitre.
• An air–fluid level in the mediastinal shadow, which is often diagnostic of the dilated oesophagus associated with achalasia.
• Aspiration pneumonia.

2 Barium swallow
This is the 'gold standard' primary investigation for dysphagia. It will direct the clinician to the level of the problem:
• Pharyngeal pouches and oesophageal webs in the upper oesophagus can be easily visualized.
• Achalasia typically shows a dilated oesophagus above a 'rat-tail' narrowing at the cardia.
• Oesophageal motility disorders can give rise to many appearances on the barium swallow, but fluoroscopic surveillance during the swallow shows muscular incoordination. Diffuse motility problems can give rise to the dramatic appearances of 'corkscrew oesophagus'.
• The appearances of a benign stricture associated with reflux or a carcinoma may be similar and endoscopy is often needed for tissue diagnosis, but the contrast study will show the clinician the length of the stricture.

3 Endoscopy
Oesophagoscopy can be used to visualize the area of the dysphagia directly and biopsies of the lesion can be taken for tissue diagnosis. However, it can be complicated by perforation, especially in the case of pharyngeal pouch, and for this reason barium studies should be the first-line investigation. Endoscopy is of little diagnostic value in motility disorders.

4 Bronchoscopy
This may be performed to look for primary carcinoma of the bronchus as a cause of the dysphagia, especially if chest radiography is abnormal.

5 Computed tomography
This is not a primary diagnostic tool, but can be useful for assessing the stage of oesophageal carcinoma (i.e. the involvement of other structures).

Oesophageal manometry and pH monitoring

These are specialist investigations. Manometry is used to assess coordination and strength of peristaltic movement in the oesophagus and also the sphincter pressures. It can be useful if other modalities have failed to show a cause for dysphagia. pH monitoring may reveal the underlying cause for a benign stricture of the oesophagus.

Fig. 9.2 Investigation and diagnosis of dysphagia.

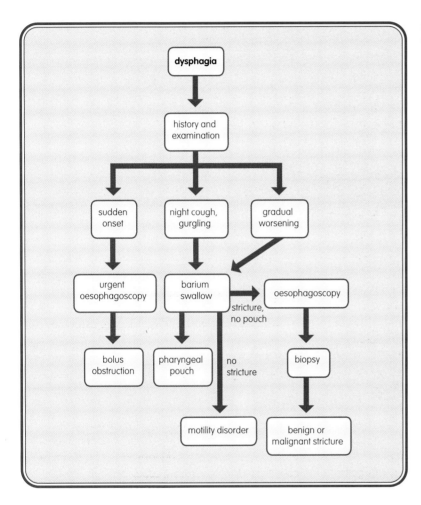

10. Breast Lump

Breast cancer is a well-publicized diagnosis and often women present with a breast lump and already have the impression that the lump is a cancer. It is important for the clinician to evaluate the lump carefully and reassure the patient without giving false hope to those who actually have a malignant tumour.

DIFFERENTIAL DIAGNOSIS OF A BREAST LUMP

The differential diagnoses are:
- Breast carcinoma.
- Fibroadenoma.
- Benign cyst.
- Fat necrosis.
- Cystosarcoma phyllodes.
- Breast abscess.
- Galactocoele.
- Duct ectasia.
- Duct papilloma.

HISTORY TO FOCUS ON THE DIFFERENTIAL DIAGNOSIS OF A BREAST LUMP

Presentation
How did the patient first become aware of the lump?
- Many lumps are incidental findings discovered while in the shower or washing and may have been present for a long time before discovery. Women who regularly examine their breasts will be more accurate in their assessment of the duration of the lump than the casual examiner.
- Some women notice asymmetry of their breasts when in front of the mirror; often they notice skin changes or dimpling and this is more suggestive of a carcinoma.
- A history of trauma preceding the discovery may alert one to the possibility of fat necrosis, but may just have been the incident that caused the discovery of a pre-existing lump.

- A lump presenting suddenly in a breastfeeding mother is likely to be a galactocoele or abscess.

Changes
How has the lump changed since its discovery?
- A lump that alters in size during the menstrual cycle is more likely to be a hormone-related benign breast change than a carcinoma.
- A lump that slowly grows in size is more likely to be a solid lump (benign or malignant), but one that doubles in size over a few days is more likely to be cystic.

Associated symptoms
Pain
Breast abscesses are acutely painful and tender.
A rapidly enlarging breast cyst may also cause pain.
Carcinomas of the breast are rarely painful (with the noticeable exception of inflammatory carcinoma).

Discharge
Ask about any discharge:
- A bloody discharge from the nipple can be a sign of malignancy, but may also be associated with benign papillomas of the duct and may also be caused by trauma during breastfeeding.
- A creamy or greenish discharge is associated with duct ectasia.
- A discharge of milky fluid with resolution of the lump in a breastfeeding mother is likely to be due to a galactocoele.

Fever
Most commonly fever is associated with an abscess, but can also be present if the patient has an inflammatory carcinoma.

Previous history
A woman who has developed a cyst or fibroadenoma is more likely to develop further cysts or fibroadenomas (but is no less likely to develop breast cancer). Similarly a past history of carcinoma should raise one's suspicions regarding any further breast lumps.

Family history

Overall a woman's risk of developing breast cancer is 1 in 11 over a lifetime. Certain genes greatly increase a woman's risk and therefore a careful history about any first or second degree relatives who have breast cancer (particularly if they developed it at an early age) should be obtained.

Drug history

Increased exposure to oestrogen is associated with an increased risk of breast cancer so a history of oral contraceptive and hormone replacement therapy usage should be taken.

Menstrual and reproductive history

Early menarche and late menopause are associated with an increased oestrogen exposure and risk of breast cancer. Breastfeeding children for more than three months seems to have some protective effects against breast cancer.

EXAMINATION OF PATIENTS WHO HAVE A BREAST LUMP

Inspection

The patient's breasts should be inspected in the seated position and any asymmetry noted. In particular certain signs are suggestive of underlying malignancy:

- Skin dimpling.
- Unilateral nipple inversion or indrawing.
- Destruction or ulceration of the nipple.
- Peau d'orange.

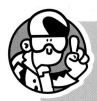

Ask the patient to identify the lump first. It may save fumbling around normal breast tissue and being unable to identify any abnormality.

Palpation

The whole of both breasts should be examined, remembering that the breast tissue extends into the axilla, and paying attention to any irregularity in the breast tissue. The characteristics of any lump (i.e. texture, mobility, and any discharge) should be carefully noted.

Texture

Hard irregular masses are characteristic of carcinoma.

Benign lumps tend to be well defined and smooth.

Cysts do not exhibit signs of fluctuance unless they are very large and lax; most cysts feel firm and can be quite difficult to distinguish from solid benign lesions.

Areas of tender nodularity, especially in the upper outer quadrants, are characteristic of benign breast change.

Mobility

Benign lumps are relatively mobile, especially fibroadenomas, which are commonly referred to as 'breast mice' because of the way they tend to dart away from under the examiner's fingers.

Any lump that is fixed to the skin or underlying muscle is malignant until proven otherwise.

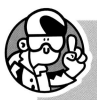

Ask the patient to push down on her hips to tense the pectoral muscles when trying to establish fixation to muscle.

Discharge

During palpation of the breast it may be possible to express some discharge from the breast. Attention should be paid to whether the discharge is coming from single or multiple ducts. The quadrant of the breast from where the discharge appears to be coming from should be carefully palpated. A small duct papilloma may be palpable in the subareolar region.

Other examination findings

Lymphadenopathy

Breast cancers spread via lymphatics draining to the axilla, supraclavicular fossa, and internal mammary chain. Axillary and supraclavicular areas should be carefully examined and the character of any palpable lymph nodes recorded.

- Malignant lymph nodes generally feel hard and craggy and may be fixed to each other or adjacent structures.
- Benign reactive lymph nodes feel soft and smooth and may be associated with inflammatory breast disease.

- With advanced malignant nodes there may be lymphoedema of the upper limb.

Hepatomegaly

Advanced carcinoma of the breast may present with liver metastases, so the size and texture of any liver edge should be noted.

INVESTIGATION OF PATIENTS WHO HAVE A BREAST LUMP

An algorithm for the investigation and diagnosis of a breast lump is given in Fig. 10.1.

Assessment of any breast lump is usually made as a three-modality investigation:

- Clinical examination.
- Radiological investigation.
- Histological examination.

This approach leads to a confident diagnosis.

Radiography

Mammography

Mammography is the investigation of choice for breast lumps in women over 35 years of age:

- Classically breast cancers appear as a spiculated dense lesion.
- Fibroadenomas and cysts tend to appear as well-defined dense lesions; long-established fibroadenomas can appear calcified.

The pattern of calcification can also give a clue about the nature of the lump:

- Well-defined coarse calcification tends to be benign.
- Malignant calcification appears powdery and is very variable in size and shape.

Ultrasonography

Breast tissue is much denser in younger women so mammography is of limited value and therefore ultrasound is used more frequently.

- Cysts appear as echo-poor well-rounded lesions.
- Fibroadenomas are well circumscribed and have internal echoes.
- Carcinomas are less well defined with irregular echoes and have characteristic acoustic shadowing behind the lesion.

Tissue sample

Fine-needle aspiration cytology

Cells of the lump can be withdrawn using a 21-gauge needle and a 10 mL syringe. The cells can be examined by the cytology department and assessed for malignancy.

Needle aspiration can also be therapeutic in the case of cysts. Benign breast cyst fluid is greenish in colour,

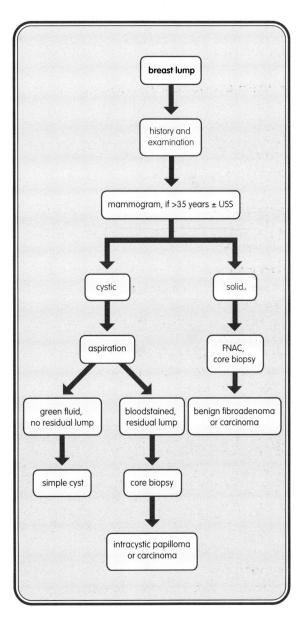

Fig. 10.1 Investigation and diagnosis of a breast lump. (FNAC, fine-needle aspiration cytology; USS, ultrasound scan.)

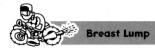

but if there is any blood staining or a residual lump the fluid should be sent for cytology.

> **If cyst aspirate is bloody or there is a residual lump further investigation is necessary.**

Wide-bore needle biopsy

Use of wide-bore/core biopsy needle allows the histologist to assess architecture, type, and differentiation of the tumour and therefore guide the surgeon in the approach to treatment.

Excision biopsy

Sometimes the diagnosis can only be truly established by diagnostic excision of the lesion, but in most cases the diagnosis is established using the biopsy techniques described above.

11. Neck Lump

Most neck pathology presents as a neck swelling. To understand neck swellings it is important to understand the basic anatomy of the neck and stuctures within each area (Fig. 11.1)

DIFFERENTIAL DIAGNOSIS OF A NECK LUMP

The differential diagnoses are:
- Midline—thyroid goitre, thyroglossal cyst, thyroid carcinoma.
- Anterior triangle of the neck—lymph node, submandibular gland tumour, branchial cyst, carotid artery aneurysm, carotid body tumour, laryngocoele, pharyngeal pouch.
- Posterior triangle—lymph node, cystic hygroma, cervical rib, subclavian artery aneurysm.
- Parotid region—parotid gland tumour, parotid calculus, parotitis.

HISTORY TO FOCUS ON THE DIFFERENTIAL DIAGNOSIS OF A NECK LUMP

General questions relating to lumps are covered in the Part II, Chapter 21.

Specific questions should cover the following.

Head and neck symptoms
Ask about pain in the mouth, nose, and sinuses. Head and neck cancers usually present with local symptoms or lymph node metastases and not generalized weight loss and malaise.

Hoarseness
This may be due to laryngeal pathology or recurrent laryngeal nerve palsy. Interference with the recurrent laryngeal nerve by a neck lump is due to direct compression and suggests a malignant infiltration, usually by thyroid cancer (due to its close relationship to this gland).

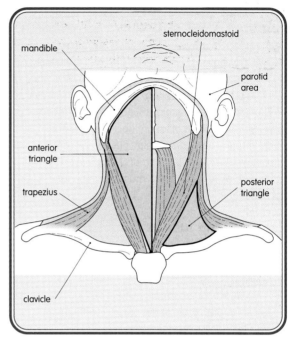

Fig. 11.1 Surface anatomy of the anterior neck.

Shortness of breath
This may be due to the lump pressing on the trachea (e.g. by a large retrosternal goitre) or the neck swelling may be due to lymphadenopathy associated with a laryngeal or bronchial malignancy as the primary cause of shortness of breath.

Dysphagia
This is discussed in Chapter 9.

Haemoptysis
A history of coughing up fresh blood may be associated with bronchial carcinoma or carcinoma of the larynx.

Weight loss
This may be associated with any malignant process of the upper gastrointestinal tract, which in turn can lead to cervical lymphadenopathy.

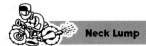
Weakness of movements of the face

This indicates involvement of the facial nerve in the underlying process. It is unusual for this to be solely due to pressure effect and usually indicates malignant infiltration of the nerve.

Features of hypo- and hyperthyroidism

Features of hyperthyroidism include nervousness or tremor, palpitations, weight loss despite increased appetite, diarrhoea, preference for cold weather, sweating, and amenorrhoea.

Features of hypothyroidism include an increase in weight, deposition of fat on the shoulders and neck, lethargy and general slowness, intolerance of cold weather, hair thinning and loss (especially outer third of the eyebrows), muscle fatigue, and constipation.

Exacerbating factors

Some lumps will only appear at certain times:

- A lump appearing behind the sternocleidomastoid on swallowing liquids may be a pharyngeal pouch.
- A laryngocoele is a small mucous outpouching that becomes prominent in the anterior triangle on coughing and sneezing.

EXAMINATION OF PATIENTS WHO HAVE A NECK LUMP

Number

Multiple neck lumps are nearly always lymph nodes.

Thorough examination of head, neck, chest, abdomen, oral cavity

Lymphadenopathy can be associated with disorders in any of these regions and they should therefore be inspected for signs of the primary condition, whether inflammatory or malignant.

Seventh cranial (facial) nerve

Full examination of the facial nerve (i.e. all major divisions) should be made if there is swelling in the parotid area to assess any invasion of the nerve by a malignant process.

Does the lump move?

Thyroid swellings typically move on swallowing. Thyroglossal cysts move on protruding the tongue.

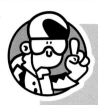

When assessing thyroid swellings, offer the patient a glass of water. It can be very difficult to swallow nothing repeatedly.

Pulsation

Is the lump pulsatile or expansile:

- Carotid aneurysms should be expansile.
- Carotid body tumours are pulsatile, but not expansile.

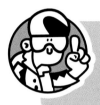

Palpate the neck from behind with the patient sitting. It is easier to position your hands in this fashion.

Eye signs

There may be occular signs of thyroid disease including:

- Retraction—the upper lid is higher than normal, but the lower lid is in normal position.
- Lid lag—the upper lid does not move at the same rate as the eye on downward gaze.
- Exophthalmos—protrusion of eyes, difficulty in convergent gaze, and loss of forehead wrinkling on upward gaze.
- Ophthalmoplegia—most commonly this affects the inferior oblique (i.e. affects looking upward and outward).
- Chemosis—oedema of the conjunctivae due to obstruction of venous and lymphatic drainage associated with increased retrobulbar pressure.

Transillumination

Cystic hygromas are found in the base of the posterior triangle and are brilliantly transilluminable. Thyroglossal cysts may also be transilluminated

INVESTIGATION OF PATIENTS WHO HAVE A NECK LUMP

An algorithm for the investigation and diagnosis of a neck lump is given in Fig. 11.2.

Special investigations

These depend upon the location of the lump and initial clinical impression.

Suspected lymphadenopathy

A series of blood tests should be performed as a routine lymphadenopathy screen including:

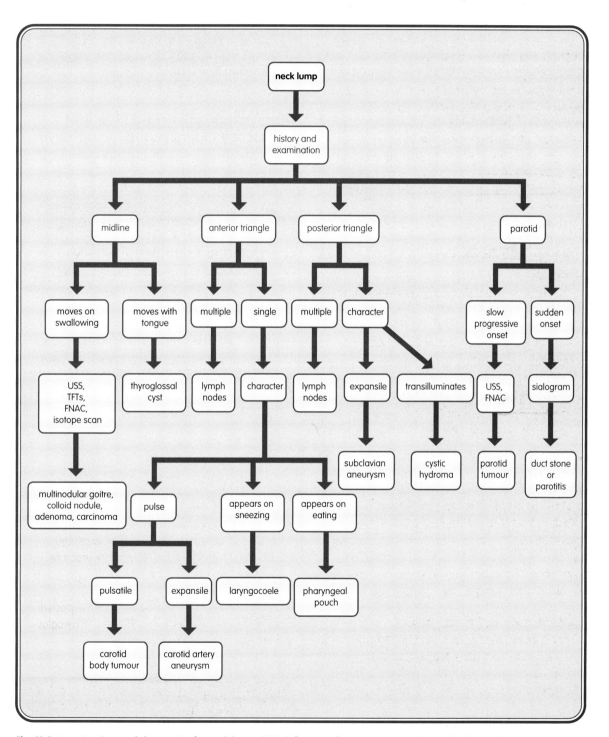

Fig. 11.2 Investigation and diagnosis of a neck lump. (FNAC, fine-needle aspiration cytology; TFTs, thyroid function tests; USS, ultrasound scan.)

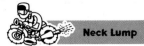

- Full blood count—anaemia may be associated with lymphoma.
- Cytomegalovirus serology—infection by this virus is associated with lymphadenopathy.
- Toxoplasma serology.
- Paul Bunnell test—for infectious mononucleosis (glandular fever due to Epstein–Barr virus infection).

Testing for human immunodeficiency virus (HIV) testing may also be considered, but only after appropriate counselling and for high-risk patients.

Thyroid swelling
Thyroid function tests are carried out to assess over- or underactivity of the gland

An ultrasound scan of the thyroid will establish the nature of the lump (i.e. whether it is solid or cystic).

Fine-needle aspiration of a solid lump can provide a diagnosis.

An isotope scan using radiolabelled pertechnate (^{99}Tc) will establish whether the lump is active thyroid tissue. The lump is usually described as 'hot' or 'cold'. Cold nodules are non-functioning thyroid areas. Carcinomas of the thyroid are usually cold nodules.

Parotid swelling
An ultrasound scan of the parotid will establish whether the swelling:

- Is cystic or solid.
- Extends deep to the facial nerve—this is important in planning surgery.

A sialogram is a contrast study of the salivary duct and will demonstrate an obstructing stone.

Mumps is a viral parotitis caused by paramyxovirus. It is bilateral in 90% of cases.

Mirror examination and fibreoptic endoscopy of larynx and hypopharynx
This may be useful to look for laryngeal and hypopharyngeal primary tumours. It is also useful to look at the vocal cord function to assess the recurrent laryngeal nerve in the case of hoarseness or as a preoperative assessment before thyroid surgery.

Computed tomography
This may be useful to assess the size and extent of neck tumours and may help to confirm the likely anatomical source of indeterminate swellings.

Barium swallow and endoscopy
These may be performed to assess pharyngeal pouch or upper oesophageal tumours. Supraclavicular fossa lymphadenopathy is classically associated with stomach carcinoma, so endoscopy may be useful to look for this condition.

12. Ischaemic Limb

Ischaemia is defined as an inadequate blood supply to an organ or limb to enable normal function. Ischaemia of a limb is often described as acute, chronic, or acute on chronic. Management and investigation depends upon the speed of onset of the symptoms.

DIFFERENTIAL DIAGNOSIS OF AN ISCHAEMIC LIMB

The differential diagnoses for acute ischaemia are:
- Embolus.
- Thrombosis.
- Trauma.

The differential diagnoses for chronic ischaemia are:
- Peripheral vascular disease (atherosclerosis).
- Buerger's disease.
- External compression (popliteal artery entrapment or thoracic outlet syndrome).
- Arteritis (e.g. systemic lupus erythematosus, Takayasu's aortitis).

HISTORY TO FOCUS ON THE DIFFERENTIAL DIAGNOSIS OF AN ISCHAEMIC LIMB

Onset and progression
The most important part of the history is how the disease presents and progresses:
- A sudden onset of severe pain, paraesthesia, and paralysis in a previously asymptomatic patient suggests an acute embolic event.
- A long history of reduced walking distance (see below) is suggestive of atherosclerotic disease (chronic ischaemia).
- A sudden worsening of symptoms in a patient who has a long history of claudication may suggest thrombosis of a critically stenosed vessel (acute on chronic ischaemia).
- The onset of pain on activity in a young patient under 30 years of age is unlikely to be due to atherosclerotic disease and more likely due to a compression or entrapment syndrome.

Claudication
Claudication is the cramping pain associated with anaerobic exercise of a muscle due to ischaemia. The pain is alleviated by rest. The severity is related to the distance walked before the onset of pain. The site at which the pain occurs gives the level of the vessel disease:
- Calf—femoropopliteal.
- Thigh—iliofemoral.
- Buttock—aortoiliac.

Rest pain
Pain at rest implies severe disease leading to ischaemia in the non-active muscle. The pain is often felt in the foot or toes. Patients will describe pain coming on at night (when the leg is elevated in bed) and relieved by resting the limb out of bed.

Previous medical history
The following conditions are associated with thromboembolic disease:
- Cerebral embolus.
- Transient ischaemic attacks.
- Amaurosis fugax.

Conditions that increase the likelihood of occlusive disease are:
- Diabetes mellitus.
- Hypertension.
- Hyperlipidaemia.

Other cardiovascular events that may be associated with an increased risk of emboli include:
- Recent myocardial infarction.
- Atrial fibrillation.

Family history
Family history of the above conditions and vascular disease is associated with an increased risk of vascular disease.

Social history
Smoking is a major risk factor in peripheral vascular disease. The risk in part is dose related, but any history of smoking is an important factor.

EXAMINATION OF PATIENTS WHO HAVE AN ISCHAEMIC LIMB

Inspection
General inspection
Chronic ischaemia can lead to:
- Hair loss.
- Ulceration.
- Blistering of the skin.

Colour
The ischaemic limb will look pale in comparison to a normal limb. Other discoloration may be seen:
- Dusky purple—deoxygenation of the tissues may give a cyanosed appearance when the limb is dependent.
- Black—necrotic patches may be seen, especially in the toes.

When assessing limbs leave both exposed for at least 5 min before comparing colour and temperature.

Other conditions, although not truly ischaemic but leading to a loss of palpable pulses peripherally, may also cause colour change:
- Blue—in deep venous thrombosis the superficial veins become engorged and a deep blue swollen limb occurs (phlegmasia cerulea dolens).
- White—a milky white limb occurs with severe oedema associated with a deep venous thrombosis (phlegmasia alba dolens) of iliofemoral veins.

Buerger's angle
The normal limb can be raised to 90 degrees without loss of colour, but an ischaemic limb will blanche on raising the limb above horizontal. The angle at which this occurs is called Buerger's angle. A Buerger's angle of less than 20 degrees indicates severe ischaemia.

After the limb has been raised the time for the colour to return can also give an indication of perfusion. In severe disease this may be over 20 s.

If the ischaemic limb is then suspended over the edge of the examination couch it will turn from white to pink and then a dusky red-purple. This is called Buerger's sign

Venous filling
In the normal limb the veins appear full when the limb is horizontal. Ischaemic limbs may have underfilled veins, which leave grooves in the skin, so-called guttering of veins. Where the veins have some filling, the angle at which they become guttered can give some idea of the degree of ischaemia.

Palpation
Temperature
The ischaemic limb will be cool in comparison to the normal limb.

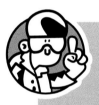

Use the back of your fingers to assess temperature. The palmar surfaces are often warm and moist and may give a false impression of temperature.

Capillary refilling
Pressure on the toe blanches the skin and the time for normal colour to return is noted. An abnormal result is more than 2 s.

Pulses
Peripheral pulses (femoral, popliteal, dorsalis pedis, and posterior tibial) must be carefully palpated, noting their presence and quality (i.e. strong, weak, or absent; see Part II, Chapter 22).

Pulses may still be palpable in the small vessel disease seen in diabetics and also in Raynaud's disease.

Aneurysm of aorta or popliteal artery
Palpate for the presence of an abdominal aortic aneurysm. Note that in thin people and those who have excessive lordosis the aorta may

be very easily palpable, but bimanual palpation either side of the aorta will indicate whether the aorta is dilated.

An easily palpable popliteal artery is usually indicative of an aneurysm. Most politeal aneurysms are bilateral and the presence of one aneurysmal popliteal artery and absence of the other popliteal pulse should alert one to the possibility of a thrombosis of the aneurysmal vessel.

Auscultation
Bruits

Listen over the femoral pulses and also in both iliac fossae for bruits, which indicate turbulent flow through a narrowed section of artery.

INVESTIGATION OF PATIENTS WHO HAVE AN ISCHAEMIC LIMB

An algorithm for the investigation and diagnosis of an ischaemic limb is given in Fig. 12.1.

Blood tests

These may include:
- Full blood count—to exclude polycythaemia as a cause of slow perfusion and thrombosis.
- Urea and electrolytes—longstanding ischaemia may lead to muscle necrosis, myoglobinaemia, and renal failure.
- Erythrocyte sedimentation rate—a marker of inflammatory vasculitic processes.

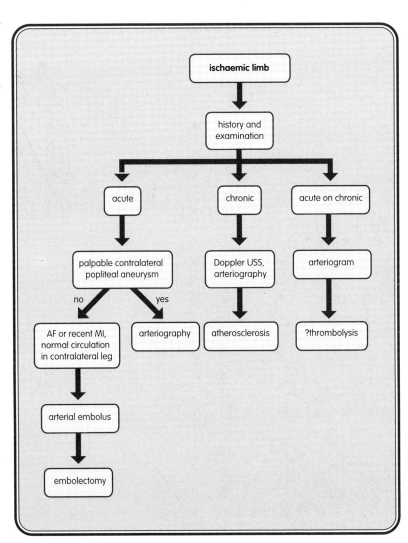

Fig. 12.1 Investigation and diagnosis of an ischaemic limb. (AF, atrial fibrillation; MI, myocardial infarction; USS, ultrasound scan.)

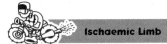

- Clotting screen—abnormalities of clotting may lead to thrombosis of venous or arterial vessels.
- Glucose—diabetic arteriopathy may be the first major complication of undiagnosed diabetes mellitus.
- Lipoproteins, triglyceride, and cholesterol—increased levels of these are associated with an increased risk of atherosclerosis.

Radiography
Chest radiography
Occlusive vessel disease is a global body disease and patients who have peripheral vascular disease are more likely to have coronary artery disease and cardiomyopathy.

Doppler ankle pressures
This is a measurement using a Doppler probe of the occlusive pressure required to stop blood flow to the ankle vessels. It is often expressed as a ratio to the brachial pressure for a comparison. It may be normal in patients who have intermittent claudication and a treadmill test may then be performed. Patients are exercised on a treadmill and have Doppler ankle pressures measured at regular intervals—a drop in pressure during the exercise is abnormal and indicates some occlusive disease.

Duplex Doppler scan
This can be used to show blood flow through vessels and can indicate the site and severity of stenoses.

Arteriography
This will demonstrate the anatomy of the vessels, any sites of stenosis, and any collateral circulation.

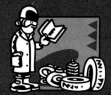

13. Leg Ulcer

An ulcer is defined as a breach in an epithelial surface. In the case of leg ulcers this is the skin.

Approximately 95% of leg ulcers are vascular in origin (either arterial or venous).

DIFFERENTIAL DIAGNOSIS OF A LEG ULCER

There are many causes of leg ulcers and they may be grouped as follows:
- Venous—varicose veins, deep vein thrombosis.
- Arterial—see Chapter 12.
- Neuropathic—diabetes mellitus, chronic alcohol abuse, other neurological disease.
- Traumatic.
- Neoplastic—squamous cell carcinoma, basal cell carcinoma, Marjolin's ulcer. = S.C.C arising in longstanding ulcer or scar
- Infectious—pyoderma gangrenosum, syphilis.
- Other—sickle cell anaemia.

HISTORY TO FOCUS ON THE DIFFERENTIAL DIAGNOSIS OF A LEG ULCER

Chronicity and progression of the ulcer should be noted and specific questions should be asked about the following.

Pain
Pain occurs in arterial, infective, and sickle cell ulcers. Neuropathic and venous ulcers are usually painless.

Venous insufficiency
A history should be taken of any deep venous thrombosis in the past as well as a history of varicose veins.

Arterial history
A detailed history of ischaemic symptoms should be obtained, including any claudication, rest pain etc. (see Chapter 12).

Trauma history
There may be a history of recent trauma to the limb. The trauma itself may have been minor, but may lead to an ulcer that is slow to heal due to underlying vascular disease that has been otherwise asymptomatic.

Bowel history
A history of altered bowel habit, especially of ulcerative colitis, may be fairly specific to pyoderma gangrenosum.

Previous medical history
This should include any history of:
- Diabetes mellitus.
- Neurological disease.
- Spinal injury.
- Coagulopathy.
- Periods of immobilization.

Social history
A detailed history should be obtained for:
- Smoking—this is associated with atherosclerotic disease.
- Alcohol intake—may lead to vitamin deficiencies and peripheral neuropathy.
- Untreated venereal disease—tertiary syphilis can lead to the development of skin ulcers and neuropathies.

EXAMINATION OF PATIENTS WHO HAVE A LEG ULCER

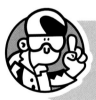

Ask the patient to stand for several minutes before assessing varicosities.

Site of the ulcer
The site may give some clues to aetiology:
- Venous ulcers occur in the lower leg, especially over the medial malleolus.

- Pressure sores and neuropathic ulcers occur over bony prominences such as the heel and malleoli.
- Arterial ulcers occur on the anterior aspect of the shin or dorsum of the foot.

Shape of the ulcer

Careful examination of the edges of the ulcer may help in diagnosis (see Chapter 18, Fig. 18.1).

Other skin changes in the limb

Arterial disease can lead to hair loss and discoloration.

Venous disease may be accompanied by varicosities, varicose eczema, haemosiderin deposits in the skin, and a unilateral swollen limb.

Inguinal lymphadenopathy may be secondary to infection or a malignant ulcer.

Arterial examination

The arteries of the lower limb should be examined (see Chapter 12 and Part II, Chapter 22).

INVESTIGATION OF PATIENTS WHO HAVE A LEG ULCER

An algorithm for the investigation and diagnosis of a leg ulcer is given in Fig. 13.1.

Blood tests

The following blood investigations may be of use:
- Full blood count—to check for anaemia and polycythaemia.
- Sickle cell test—in Afro-Caribbean patients to exclude sickle cell disease or trait.
- Glucose—to exclude undiagnosed diabetes mellitus.
- Erythrocyte sedimentation rate—to check for vasculitis.
- Antibody screen—to exclude vasculitis.
- Venereal disease research laboratory (VDRL) test —for suspected syphilis.

Culture swab

The organism responsible for an infective ulcer may be cultured in the microbiology laboratory. Most ulcers are colonized by bacteria and so the results must be interpreted with due consideration.

Arterial investigations

If arterial disease is suspected investigations (as detailed in Chapter 12) should be carried out.

Venography and ultrasonography

These may be performed to assess the patency of the deep venous system as well as demonstrate the existence of incompetent valves leading to varicose veins.

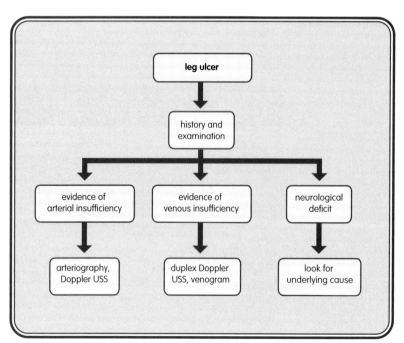

Fig. 13.1 Investigation and diagnosis of a leg ulcer. (USS, ultrasound scan.)

Biopsy of ulcer

Suspected malignancy should be investigated by biopsy of the lesion. Longstanding venous ulcers can undergo malignant change (Marjolin's ulcer) and so the edges of these should be biopsied too.

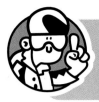

Any suspicious ulcers should be biopsied to exclude malignancy.

Shape of ulcer + ass. dx.

(1) Sloping: venous ulcer/healing traumatic ulcer

(2) Punched out: Trophic ulcer (=?)
          Neuropathic ulcer

(3) Undermined = P. sores/TB ulcer

(4) Rolled edge = BCC

(5) Everted edge = SCC

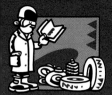

14. Groin Swelling

Swelling in the groin is one of the most common presenting complaints in the general surgical outpatient clinic, and to a lesser degree as a surgical emergency.

> An irreducible femoral hernia may appear suddenly with no past history of a hernia.

DIFFERENTIAL DIAGNOSIS OF A GROIN SWELLING

The differential diagnoses of a groin swelling are:
- Inguinal hernia. *→ above + medial to pubic tubercle*
- Femoral hernia. *→ below + lateral to pubic tubercle.*
- Lymphadenopathy.
- Hydrocoele of cord.
- Femoral artery aneurysm.
- Saphena varix.
- Lipoma or other adnexal mass.
- Psoas bursa or abscess.
- Undescended or retractile testis.

HISTORY TO FOCUS ON THE DIFFERENTIAL DIAGNOSIS OF A GROIN SWELLING

The patient usually presents to the general practitioner because he or she has discovered a lump, but occasionally a hernia is an incidental finding. In either scenario several important questions about the lump should be asked during the routine history

How did the lump first appear?
A history of sudden appearance of the lump following lifting or straining is usually a good indication that the lump may be a hernia, although the event in question may have just brought the lump to the patient's attention.

Is the lump present all the time?
Uncomplicated hernias and saphena varix may disappear on lying down. Incarcerated or irreducible hernias are present all the time as are other swellings in the differential diagnosis list (see above).

Any associated symptoms?
If the lump is lymphadenopathy it may be associated with general malaise, a flu-like illness, or recent skin infection. If malaise is severe and associated with anorexia, vomiting, and colicky abdominal pain suspect an incarcerated or even strangulated hernia.

Is the lump painful?
Characteristic pain patterns include the following:
- Sudden onset of a tender irreducible hernia suggests that the hernia is strangulated.
- Colicky abdominal pain with vomiting and distension may indicate intestinal obstruction.
- Sudden severe pain and generalized abdominal pain may indicate peritonitis resulting from a strangulated hernia.
- Lymphadenopthy can be very tender, but does not usually cause pain at rest
- Pain on hip extension may be associated with psoas abscess, but may be due to direct pressure of enlarged lymph nodes.

Direct questioning
Underlying causes of hernias include any cause of increased abdominal pressure such as:
- Straining to pass urine.
- Constipation.
- History of a chronic cough.
- Heavy manual labour.

There may be a history of lower limb trauma producing ascending infection and lymphadenopathy.

EXAMINATION OF PATIENTS WHO HAVE A GROIN SWELLING

General examination

Examination should include the whole of the abdomen, looking for abdominal masses and ascites. Remember to examine the perineum and rectum. Anal tumours may give rise to lymphadenopathy in the groins and prostatic enlargement may be the underlying cause for hernias.

Examination of the lump

The groins should be examined when the patient is standing and lying down. The characteristics of the different lumps in the differential diagnosis are as follows.

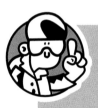

Always examine the patient lying and standing. Hernias, saphena varix and varicoceles may become prominent only on standing.

Inguinal hernia

The swelling appears through the external inguinal ring. It has a cough impulse and is compressible. It appears above and medial to the pubic tubercle and does not transilluminate.

Femoral hernia

This has the same characteristics as the inguinal hernia, but the bulge lies below the inguinal ligament. It emerges below and lateral to the pubic tubercle and is not tender except in the presence of strangulation.

Lymphadenopathy

The groin lymph nodes lie below the inguinal ligament. They are usually firm and rubbery with normal overlying skin. The lower limb and perineum should be carefully inspected to look for an infective or malignant cause.

Hydrocele of the cord

This is a smooth rounded swelling that moves on gentle traction of the testis. It is possible to get above the swelling on examination and the swelling is not reducible, but does transilluminate.

Femoral artery aneurysm

The main feature of a femoral artery aneurysm is an expansile swelling in the groin. Pulsatility alone may be present in prevascular femoral hernia or lymphadenopathy.

Saphena varix

A saphena varix is only present on standing. It has a cough impulse or fluid thrill and is compressible and refills. Tapping on the long saphenous vein below the varix produces a fluid thrill.

Undescended and retractile testis

The characteristic feature here is an empty hemiscrotum on the ipsilateral side. Retractile testes can be milked down into the scrotum, but this is rarely possible for undescended testes.

INVESTIGATION OF PATIENTS WHO HAVE A GROIN SWELLING

An algorithm for the investigation and diagnosis of a groin swelling is given in Fig. 14.1. Usually the diagnosis has been established by a careful history and examination. Some specialized investigations may help in equivocal cases to establish the diagnosis.

Herniography

Sometimes the patient gives a good history of a hernia, but when he or she presents for examination there is little to find. Herniography involves injecting water-soluble contrast into the peritoneal cavity and attempting to visualize the hernial defect by running the contrast into the hernia sac.

Doppler duplex scan

This may be useful for demonstrating saphenofemoral incompetence in the case of a saphena varix

Lymphadenopathy screen

Screening for an underlying cause of lymphadenopathy includes:
- Full blood count.
- Serology for antibodies to cytomegalovirus, and *Toxoplasma gondii.*
- Paul–Bunnell or monospot test to detect heterophil antibodies in Epstein–Bunnell infection (infectious mononucleosis).

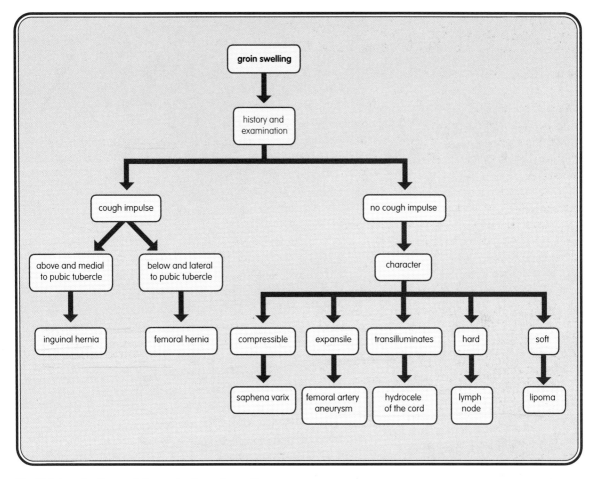

Fig. 14.1 Investigation and diagnosis of a groin swelling.

15. Scrotal Swelling

Scrotal swellings are another very common presentation to the surgical outpatient department and to the acute surgical emergency department.

DIFFERENTIAL DIAGNOSIS OF A SCROTAL SWELLING

The differential diagnoses are:
- Inguinoscrotal hernia.
- Epididymal cyst.
- Hydrocoele of the cord.
- Haematocele.
- Varicocele.
- Epididymo-orchitis.
- Testicular tumour.
- Testicular torsion.

HISTORY TO FOCUS ON THE DIFFERENTIAL DIAGNOSIS OF A SCROTAL SWELLING

Age
The patient's age may be of some help in diagnosis. It is rare for testicular torsion to present in men over 30 years of age. Testicular tumours also occur in particular age groups:
- Teratomas occur in younger men (age 20–30 years).
- Seminomas usually present in older men (aged 30–50 years).

Pain
Most scrotal swellings give rise to discomfort as a result of compression by clothes, but pain is not usually a feature of epididymal cysts, hydroceles, tumours, or varicoceles.

Inguinal hernias can cause moderate discomfort on straining.

Pain is the main feature in testicular torsion and epididymo-orchitis:
- Testicular torsion gives rise to severe scrotal pain of sudden onset and it may be associated with vomiting and suprapubic pain. There may be some preceding episodes of similar but less severe pain due to incomplete torsion due to the underlying anatomical abnormality (Fig 15.1)
- Epididymo-orchitis usually has a longer more insidious onset and usually there is no history of preceding testicular pain.

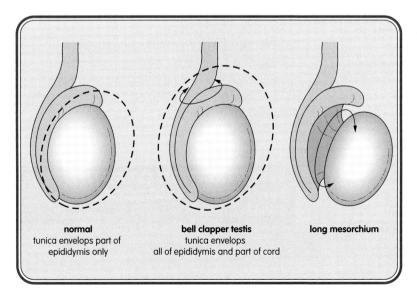

Fig. 15.1 Abnormalities leading to torsion of the testis.

normal
tunica envelops part of epididymis only

bell clapper testis
tunica envelops all of epididymis and part of cord

long mesorchium

Always check the testes of adolescent boys who complain of lower abdominal pain—it may be due to torsion.

A varicocele is a common case in examinations. The patient will be lying on the bed when you are asked to examine his scrotum. Stand the patient up before starting your examination. The diagnosis will be easy and you will score points for correct technique.

Any history of trauma?

Scrotal trauma is usually well remembered by the patient and often occurs in sporting injuries. A history of sudden painful swelling after such injury is often indicative of a haematocele.

Any micturition problems?

Epididymo-orchitis is usually associated with urinary tract infection and there may therefore be a preceding or concomitant history of dysuria and frequency. This may be absent in viral epididymo-orchitis.

EXAMINATION OF PATIENTS WHO HAVE A SCROTAL SWELLING

The scrotal swelling should be examined when the patient is standing up.

Character of swelling

Testicular tumours are usually hard non-tender swellings that usually occupy the whole testis by the time the patient presents to the clinician.

Hydroceles and haematoceles are usually much softer and fluctuant, but in a chronic haematocele where the blood has clotted, the appearance can be very similar to that of a testicular tumour.

Varicoceles are not palpable in the supine patient, but on standing have a characteristic feel that is often described as 'a bag of worms'.

In torsion of the testis the testis lies horizontally and is exquisitely tender.

The scrotal skin may also be changed. Epididymo-orchitis can give rise to a red swollen scrotum, but this may also occur with prolonged torsion or advanced testicular tumour.

Is it possible to palpate above the swelling?

Inguinal hernias descending in the scrotum can be easily identified because it is impossible to get above the swelling. All other swellings are confined to the scrotum.

Is the swelling separate from the testis and epididymis?

This is an important diagnostic feature:
- Epididymal cysts are palpable within the epididymis and separate from the testis.
- Encysted hydroceles of the cord are also palpable separately from the testis and epididymis.
- The testis is not usually palpable within a vaginal hydrocele or haematocele, but occasionally the surface of the testis can be felt in a lax hydrocele.
- The testis is palpable through a varicocele and if the patient is laid flat the scrotal contents feel normal.

Is the swelling transilluminable?

Placing a torch behind the swelling may produce a glow in the whole swelling. If this occurs it is indicative of clear fluid in the swelling, as occurs with hydroceles and epididymal cysts. Haematoceles are not transilluminable.

INVESTIGATION OF PATIENTS WHO HAVE A SCROTAL SWELLING

An algorithm for the investigation and diagnosis of a scrotal swelling is given in Fig. 15.2.

Several basic investigations may be useful adjuncts to the clinical examination.

Urinalysis

This establishes the presence of any underlying urinary infection if there is epididymo-orchitis and can guide antibiotic therapy. It may also establish an infective cause for a secondary hydrocele.

Ultrasonography

This is a useful investigation for examining the testis and epididymis. This is especially important if there is a hydrocele or haematocele where the testis is not clearly palpable. It may establish a cause for a secondary hydrocele.

Specialist ultrasound with Doppler colour flow can establish whether the blood flow to the testis is

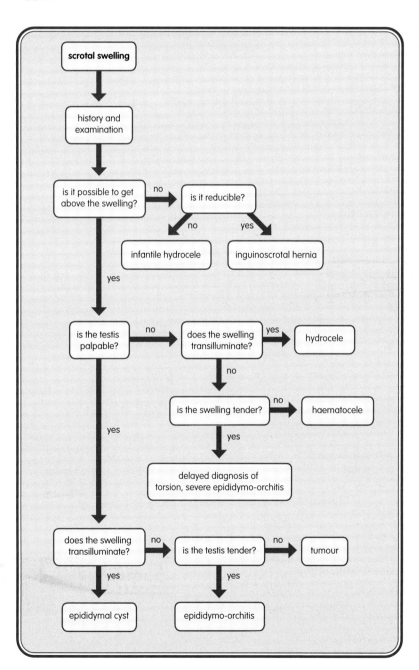

Fig. 15.2 Investigation and diagnosis of a scrotal swelling.

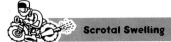

normal and therefore help in the diagnosis of torsion (but see below).

β-human chorionic gonadotrophin and α-fetoprotein

These tumour markers may be increased in the presence of testicular tumour.

Operative exploration

The differential diagnosis of epididymo-orchitis and torsion can be very difficult clinically and even Doppler ultrasound is not a foolproof way for distinguishing one from the other. It is therefore often wise to explore the acutely painful testis, especially in the young patient. Suspected torsion is a surgical emergency.

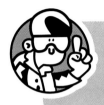
'A scar in the scrotum is better than only one testis in the scrotum'. If in doubt explore a painful testis.

16. Haematuria

Haematuria is the passage of blood in the urine and can be either:

- Macroscopic ('frank')—visible to the naked eye.
- Microscopic—detectable only with urine testing sticks or microscope examination.

Other pigments may discolour the urine giving the appearance of haematuria, including drug therapies (e.g. co-danthramer) or vegetable pigments (e.g. beetroot). The urine dipstick also picks up myoglobin and may show a positive reaction in muscle trauma.

It is useful to think of the causes of haematuria in terms of anatomy (Fig. 16.1).

DIFFERENTIAL DIAGNOSIS OF SURGICAL CAUSES OF HAEMATURIA

The differential diagnosis of haematuria can be considered in terms of the parts of the genitourinary tract involved as follows:

- Kidney—calculus, transitional cell carcinoma, adenocarcinoma, trauma, pyelonephritis.
- Ureter—ureteric calculus, transitional cell carcinoma.
- Bladder—transitional cell carcinoma, cystitis, calculus.
- Prostate and urethra—prostatitis, trauma.

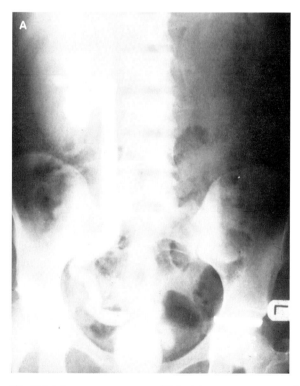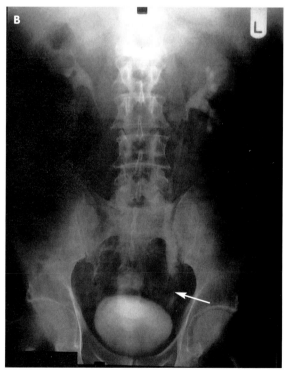

Fig. 16.1 Intravenous urograms. **(A)** An intravenous urogram showing right hydronephrosis and hydroureter. **(B)** An intravenous urogram showing a filling defect in the left lower ureter (arrow) due to ureteric carcinoma.

Never insert a suprapubic catheter into someone who has haematuria of undiagnosed cause. It may be due to a bladder tumour, which may be seeded into the abdominal wall by the catheter.

HISTORY TO FOCUS ON THE DIFFERENTIAL DIAGNOSIS OF HAEMATURIA

Pain

Painless haematuria is often associated with urothelial tumours of bladder, ureter, or kidney.

The characteristics of pain associated with haematuria may suggest the diagnosis:

- Painful micturition indicates inflammation of the bladder or prostate.
- Colicky loin to groin pain is typical of a ureteric calculus.
- Burning pain in the penis or urethral opening in women is associated with urinary infection.
- Pain in the perineum associated with dysuria, fever, and rigors is seen in prostatitis.
- Constant dull loin pain can be a sign of renal carcinoma.

Clots

Spindle-shaped clots are usually seen in renal bleeding (e.g. due to renal carcinoma).

Large clots in the urine indicate bladder pathology.

Drug history

Oral anticoagulants are an important cause of haematuria:

- Minor bleeding may become quite frank haematuria when the patient takes warfarin.
- Overanticoagulation can present with frank haematuria.

EXAMINATION OF PATIENTS WHO HAVE HAEMATURIA

Abdominal examination

The examination includes a general abdominal examination, but specific features should be looked for.

Bladder

It is unusual for a bladder tumour to be large enough to palpate abdominally, but the bladder itself may be enlarged secondary to urinary retention due to infection or clot obstruction of urinary flow.

Renal mass

Renal tumours may be palpable on bimanual examination and ballotting.

Rectal examination

The prostate is easily palpable on rectal examination:

- An exquisitely tender prostate is a feature of prostatitis.
- In perineal trauma where the membranous urethra has been ruptured the prostate rides high.
- A smooth enlarged prostate is benign.
- A hard craggy prostate is probably malignant.

INVESTIGATION OF PATIENTS WHO HAVE HAEMATURIA

An algorithm for the investigation and diagnosis of haematuria is given in Fig. 16.2.

Urine dipstick

This will show minute traces of blood in the urine. It will also indicate the presence of protein and nitrites from bacterial breakdown of urea, suggesting infection.

Microscopy and culture

Microscopy will confirm the presence of red blood cells and will also reveal the presence of white cells and organisms in infection. Culture of the urine will confirm the identity of the organism and help to identify the antibiotic sensitivity.

Urine cytology

Urothelial tumours will shed cells into the urine that can be seen on staining and microscopy.

Early morning specimens of urine (EMUs) have a higher yield of cells and so patients should be asked to provide the first specimen of the day for cytology.

Blood tests
Full blood count
This may reveal:
- Anaemia in severe haematuria.
- Polycythaemia in renal carcinoma (due to erythropoietin secretion).

Urea and electrolytes
These will indicate any degree of renal failure. Remember that renal failure will not occur until 60% of kidney function is lost and therefore normal urea and creatinine levels do not indicate that there is no renal damage.

Plain radiography and contrast studies
Approximately 90% of kidney stones are radio-opaque and will show up on a plain abdominal film (KUB is used to refer to a plain film showing the kidneys, ureter, and bladder.)

Radiolucent stones will show up on an intravenous urogram (IVU), which will reveal delayed excretion or dilatation of collecting systems and so indicate any obstruction.

Ultrasound scan
Ultrasound scans show:
- Dilatation of the collecting systems.
- Intrarenal pathology such as tumours or stones.

Cystoscopy and biopsy
Direct examination of the urethra and bladder can reveal the pathology causing haematuria such as a bladder tumour.

Retrograde contrast studies of the ureters can also be performed by cystoscopic insertion of ureteric catheters. Such investigations can reveal small urothelial tumours of the ureters.

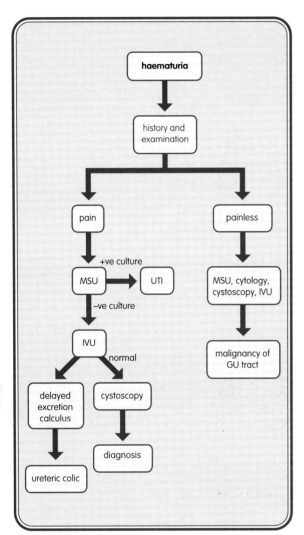

Fig. 16.2 Investigation and diagnosis of haematuria. (GU, genitourinary; IVU, intravenous urogram; MSU, mid-stream urine; UTI, urinary tract infection.)

17. Urinary Difficulty

Urinary difficulty is a very common problem in the aging population and may be tolerated as part of 'old age' by many for several years before seeking medical help. Often the patient does not present until he or she (most people who have urinary difficulty are male) cannot pass urine at all (i.e. they have urinary retention).

Chronic urinary retention, where the bladder has not completely emptied for a long time, can cause renal failure.

DIFFERENTIAL DIAGNOSIS OF URINARY DIFFICULTY

The differential diagnoses are:
- Benign prostatic hypertrophy.
- Prostate cancer.
- Bladder neck and urethral obstruction: primary or secondary (e.g. due to stricture, carcinoma, calculus).
- Pelvic mass in women (e.g. uterine tumour).
- Cystocele in women (e.g. due to anterior vaginal wall collapse).
- Neurological causes.
- Constipation.

HISTORY TO FOCUS ON THE DIFFERENTIAL DIAGNOSIS OF URINARY DIFFICULTY

Symptoms
The symptoms of urinary difficulty can be broadly split into obstructive and instability:
- Obstructive symptoms are hesitancy, poor stream, postmicturition dribbling, and a sensation of incomplete voiding.
- Detrusor instability symptoms are urgency, urge incontinence, frequency, and nocturia.

Often these symptoms are mixed in obstructive disease because chronic obstruction leads to detrusor hypertrophy and instability. Further history should then be obtained to find the cause of the pathology.

Penile discharge
Urethritis is often associated with stricture formation (gonorrhoea in particular causes stricture in the bulbous urethra after infection of the periurethral glands) and subsequent micturition problems.

The passage of frank blood through the urethra following perineal trauma is suggestive of urethral injury.

Backache
A history of unrelenting back pain and sciatica may be indicative of metastatic deposits in the spine as may be seen in prostatic carcinoma. It may also predate neurological urinary difficulty in cauda equina syndrome.

Radiotherapy
Previous radiotherapy (e.g. for a rectal tumour) can lead to a radiation cystitis.

Instrumentation
Damage from instrumentation may have occurred at a previous operation to the bladder or prostate or result from a traumatic catheterization or self-inflicted trauma.

Trauma
Low back injury may cause compression of the sacral roots causing cauda equina syndrome.

A history of a fall astride a bar or pole should alert the clinician to the possibility of membranous urethral injury. Any patient who has such a history leading to retention should not be catheterized urethrally. Specialist investigation should be performed under the supervision of the urology team (see below).

Drug history
Any drug that has anticholinergic side effects will affect bladder emptying, the most common drugs being tricyclic antidepressants and propantheline.

EXAMINATION OF PATIENTS WHO HAVE URINARY DIFFICULTY

General examination

Longstanding urinary difficulties can interfere with renal function and such patients may be uraemic. The clinician should look for:

- Anaemia.
- A lemon tinge to the skin.
- Furred tongue.
- A uraemic smell.

Abdominal examination

The most obvious feature in obstructive urinary problems is bladder distension. The bladder may be palpated as a smooth mass arising out of the pelvis and is dull to percussion. Renal enlargement may be present in longstanding obstructive uropathy.

Digital rectal examination

The prostate is easily felt through the rectal mucosa and its character should be noted.

Benign features include smoothness, firmness, and preservation of the median sulcus.

Malignant characteristics include:

- A hard craggy gland.
- A discrete hard nodule.
- Loss of the median sulcus.
- Fixity or erosion through rectal mucosa.

Vaginal examination

This should be performed in women to exclude a pelvic mass.

Neurological examination

If there is any history of back injury or pain a neurological examination of the lower limbs and perineum should be performed to elicit any deficit, especially in the sacral dermatomes. A deficit in this distribution may suggest cauda equina syndrome.

INVESTIGATION OF PATIENTS WHO HAVE URINARY DIFFICULTY

An algorithm for the investigation and diagnosis of urinary difficulty is given in Fig. 17.1.

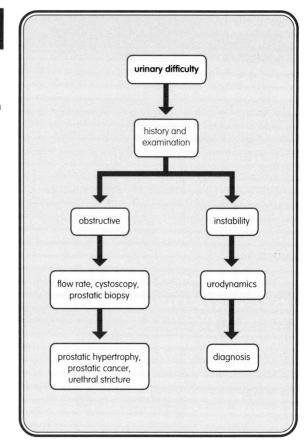

Fig. 17.1 Investigation and diagnosis of urinary difficulty.

Urine dipstick, culture, and microscopy

Urine should be sent for analysis to rule out infective causes. Cytology may also be useful (see Chapter 16).

Blood tests
Full blood count

This may show anaemia associated with chronic renal failure. An increased white cell count can indicate underlying infection.

Urea and electrolytes

These are measured to assess renal function.

Prostate-specific antigen

This may be increased in prostatic carcinoma, but can also be falsely increased in prostatitis or after urethral catheterization.

Flow rate

This is a simple test to measure the flow of urine. Obstructive pathology causes a low flow rate and prolonged voiding time.

A poor flow rate may be due to passage of a small volume of urine. The patient must pass over 100 mL of urine to obtain an acurate flow rate recording.

Urodynamics

This usually incorporates a flow test as above, but also measures bladder pressures using a special catheter. It can demonstrate bladder instability and hypersensitive bladders.

Radiography

Plain abdominal radiography—a KUB view (i.e. showing kidneys, ureters, and bladder)—can show urinary calculi.

A contrast study (intravenous urography) may show:

- Renal tract dilatation.
- A prostatic impression on the cystogram phase.
- Trabeculation of the bladder wall.
- Postmicturition residual urine.
- Radiolucent stones.

Ultrasonography

As well as showing renal tract dilatation ultrasound may also demonstrate the prostate, bladder wall thickening, and residual urine volume.

Cystoscopy

This is the best investigation to show obstructive lesions of the urethra, prostate, and bladder neck.

Ascending urethrography

Where there has been a fall astride an object and urethral damage is a possibility, water-soluble contrast may be gently injected into the urethra under fluoroscopic surveillance to ensure that there is no urethral injury before catheterization.

18. Skin Lesion

Skin lesions are a common presentation at surgical outpatients and they can range from being non-significant to being life-threatening. It is therefore of paramount importance to be able to distinguish between these lesions.

DIFFERENTIAL DIAGNOSIS OF A SKIN LESION

It is helpful to consider the lesions in terms of anatomical layers. The differential diagnoses of a skin lesion are:
- Ulcers—arterial, venous, vasculitic, pressure, malignant, neuropathic.
- In the skin—melanoma, benign naevus, viral wart, seborrhoeic keratosis, strawberry naevus, telangectasia, pyogenic granuloma, dermoid cyst, sebaceous cyst, neurofibroma, keloid, hypertrophic scar.
- Under the skin—lipoma, arteriovenous malformation, ganglion, lymph node, bursa, implantation dermoid.

HISTORY TO FOCUS ON THE DIFFERENTIAL DIAGNOSIS OF A SKIN LESION

How was it discovered?
Many skin lumps are noted while washing and may have been present for some time. There may be a history of local penetrating trauma preceding the lump alerting the clinician to the possibility of a foreign body. The lump may have presented because of pain.

Duration and development of symptoms
The duration of a lump may provide some clues about its nature:
- A lump that has been present for years is more likely to be a benign condition.
- A rapidly growing lesion of short duration is more suggestive of a malignant lesion.
- Cystic lesions can grow rapidly and cause pain if they become infected.

Change in size and shape
How a lump changes in time may also be helpful in diagnosis. A rapidly growing lesion may ulcerate the skin and rapid change may be a feature of malignancy.

Itching and bleeding
These are both worrying symptoms in a pigmented lesion and are often associated with malignancy, especially malignant melanoma.

Previous lesions
The patient may have had previous lesions excised. This is of particular importance in malignant melanoma.

EXAMINATION OF PATIENTS WHO HAVE A SKIN LESION

Lump
Position, size, shape, colour, texture edge, and composition of the lesion should be recorded (see Part II, Chapter 22).
Specific features may be elicited as outlined below

Position
Most lesions can occur anywhere on the body, but some have a preponderance for certain areas of the body:
- Warts—most common on the palmar surface of the hands or on the feet (i.e. verruca).
- Seborrhoeic keratosis—not on areas subject to abrasion.
- Moles—more often on limbs.
- Malignant melanoma—limbs, head, and neck.
- Strawberry naevus—usually head and neck.
- Hydradenitis suppurativa—axilla and groin.
- Basal cell carcinoma—upper one-third of the face and forehead.

Surface
Note the surface of the lesion:
- Smooth—any subcutaneous lesion, sebaceous cyst, dermoid cyst.

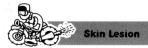

- Pearly—early basal cell carcinoma.
- Rough—viral wart, papilloma, seborrhoeic keratosis.

Lymph drainage

Lymph nodes may be enlarged in:
- Malignant melanoma—often infiltrated with tumour.
- Squamous cell carcinoma—two-thirds will be enlarged because of malignant infiltration, one-third will be enlarged because of infection of the tumour.
- Pyogenic granuloma—local nodes are only enlarged if there is severe infection.

Local tissues

Melanoma may exhibit a depigmented halo or satellite nodules.

Squamous cell carcinoma may produce a thickened oedematous local reaction.

Special features

Some lesions have pathognomonic features:
- Seborrhoeic keratosis—can be picked off leaving a pink patch of skin with a few capillary bleeding points only.
- Strawberry naevus—is compressible and the lesion can be completely emptied of blood leaving a baggy patch of skin, which gradually refills on releasing pressure.
- Arteriovenous malformation—may have a thrill or bruit and can be associated with a giant limb.
- Aneurysm—is pulsatile and expansile.

Ulcers

The edges of the ulcer are the most revealing feature of the underlying cause (Fig 18.1).

INVESTIGATION OF PATIENTS WHO HAVE A SKIN LESION

An algorithm for the investigation and diagnosis of a skin lesion is given in Fig. 18.2.

Often the diagnosis is made from the history and examination.

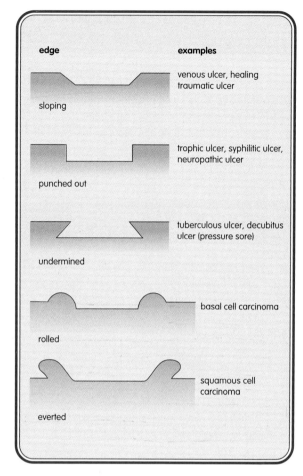

Fig. 18.1 Types of ulcer and typical examples.

Excision biopsy

The only investigation of importance is histology and this is usually performed as an excision biopsy under local anaesthetic. Occasionally incisional wedge biopsies are taken of large lesions and further treatment is planned when definitive histology is available.

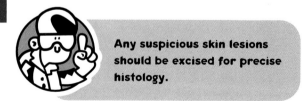

Any suspicious skin lesions should be excised for precise histology.

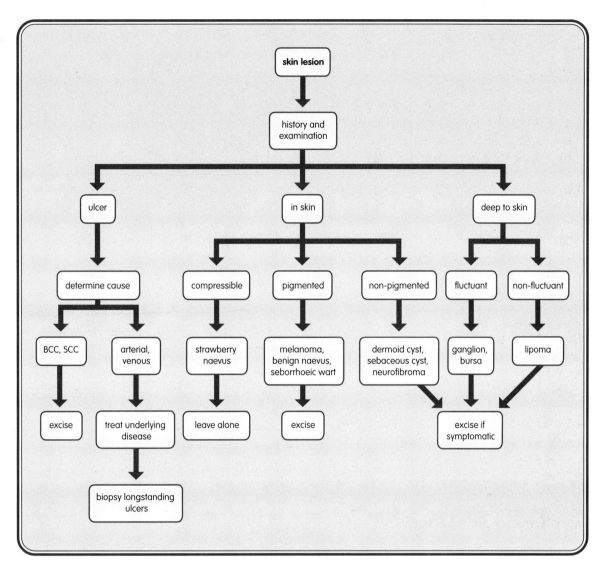

Fig. 18.2 Investigation and diagnosis of a skin lesion. (BCC, basal cell carcinoma; SCC, squamous cell carcinoma.)

19. Anaemia

Anaemia results from many chronic diseases. In this chapter we will be concerned only with the direct causes of anaemia that are relevant to the general surgeon.

DIFFERENTIAL DIAGNOSIS OF ANAEMIA

It is useful to divide up the anaemias into types depending upon cell size.

Microcytic hypochromic anaemia results from blood loss from the gastrointestinal or genitourinary tracts and inadequate iron intake or absorption.

Normochromic anaemia is a feature of chronic disease (e.g. chronic renal failure, rheumatoid arthritis).

Macrocytic anaemia is caused by vitamin B_{12} or folate deficiency, which may be secondary to:

- Pernicious anaemia—an autoimmune condition in which there are autoantibodies to gastric parietal cells or intrinsic factor and as a result vitamin B_{12} cannot be absorbed.
- Anaemia following gastrectomy.
- Anaemia in coeliac disease.
- Anaemia following ileal resection or occurring with ileal disease (e.g. Crohn's disease).
- Anaemia due to alcoholic liver disease.

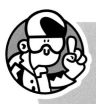

Anaemia is a symptom and not a diagnosis. The underlying cause should be found.

HISTORY TO FOCUS ON THE DIFFERENTIAL DIAGNOSIS OF ANAEMIA

Symptoms
The following symptoms are common for all causes of anaemia:

- Fatigue.
- Headaches.
- Lightheadedness.
- Breathlessness (especially on effort).
- Angina.
- Intermittent claudication.
- Palpitations.

However, their severity is not only related to the degree of anaemia, but also to its speed of onset. A slow gradual anaemia will be well tolerated down to very low haemoglobin levels, but a rapid blood loss may produce some profound symptoms.

Gastrointestinal blood loss
A careful history about possible gastrointestinal loss of blood should be obtained. Symptoms include:

- Dyspepsia.
- Haematemesis—due to peptic ulceration, oesophagitis, or gastric or oesophageal cancer.
- Melaena—due to peptic ulceration, oesophagitis, or gastric or oesophageal cancer.
- Fresh rectal blood loss—due to carcinoma of the colon or rectum or inflammatory bowel disease.
- Change in bowel habit—due to carcinoma of the colon or rectum or inflammatory bowel disease.

These symptoms (especially the rectal blood loss) may be very mild, but over a long time can produce profound anaemia.

Common causes of asymptomatic blood loss from the gastrointestinal tract are peptic ulceration and caecal carcinoma.

Menstrual history
A history of the following may be sufficient to cause chronic anaemia in premenopausal women:

- Heavy periods (menorrhagia).
- Intermenstrual bleeding.

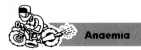

Family history

A family history of various conditions may be very informative. Such conditions include:

- Coeliac disease.
- Familial polyposis coli and carcinoma of the colon.
- Bleeding diatheses.
- Haemoglobinopathies.

Drug history

Several drugs may lead to gastrointestinal blood loss including:

- Non-steroidal anti-inflammatory drugs.
- Corticosteroids.
- Potassium supplements.

Drugs that cause bone marrow suppression include:

- Cytotoxic drugs
- Chloramphenicol.

Other drugs cause anaemia by causing folate depletion. These drugs include phenytoin, primidone and methotrexate.

Alcohol

As well a being a risk factor for upper gastrointestinal haemorrhage, alcohol is also associated with chronic liver disease.

Travel

The commonest cause of anaemia worldwide is hookworm infestation of the gastrointestinal tract. Tropical sprue may be another acquired condition leading to anaemia.

EXAMINATION OF PATIENTS WHO HAVE ANAEMIA

General examination

The degree of anaemia can be estimated by looking at the colour of the conjunctivae and mucous membranes.

There may be signs of weight loss and cachexia associated with either malignancy or chronic inflammatory bowel disease.

Cardiovascular system

The following are features of anaemia of any cause:

- Rapid and bounding pulse.
- A systolic flow murmur.

- If anaemia is severe there may be a degree of heart failure.

Mouth

Pale mucous membranes are a non-specific sign of anaemia, but certain features in the mouth may be associated with specific causes:

- Smooth tongue—due to atrophy of papillae is seen in iron deficiency.
- Angular stomatitis—may be present with either iron deficiency or vitamin B_{12} deficiency.
- Glossitis—inflamed tongue seen in vitamin B_{12} deficiency and may also be seen in iron deficiency anaemia with dysphagia or as part of Plummer–Vinson syndrome.
- Telangectasia on lips—associated with Osler–Weber–Rendu syndrome and pigmentation associated with Peutz–Jeghers syndrome.

Skin and adnexa

There may be skin pigmentation changes:

- Lemon-yellow tint in vitamin B_{12} deficiency.
- Vitiligo occurs in patients who have pernicious anaemia.

Hair and nails may be affected in iron deficiency anaemia resulting in:

- Brittle hair.
- Brittle nails.
- Koilonychia—spoon-shaped nails.

Abdominal examination

Palpable features in the abdomen that may be associated with iron deficiency anaemia include:

- Tumour of large bowel—especially caecum.
- Fibroid uterus.
- Gastric carcinoma.
- Inflammatory mass due to Crohn's disease.

Examination of the abdomen should include rectal examination for rectal tumours and melaena stool, and a vaginal examination as well in women.

INVESTIGATION OF PATIENTS WHO HAVE ANAEMIA

An algorithm for the investigation and diagnosis of anaemia is given in Fig. 19.1.

Blood tests
Full blood count
This will tell the clinician the degree and type of anaemia.

Reticulocyte count
This reflects the number of immature red cells being produced by the bone marrow. The reticulocyte count is increased in haemolytic anaemias.

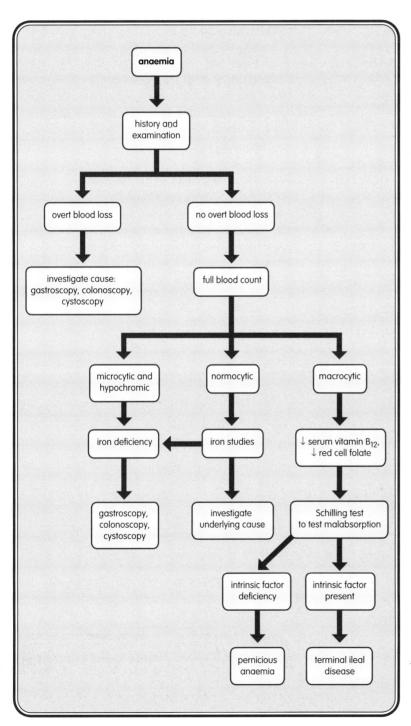

Fig. 19.1 Investigation and diagnosis of anaemia.

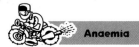

Iron studies

Iron studies may help distinguish between iron deficiency and chronic disease anaemias:

- Serum iron level is low in both iron deficiency and anaemia of chronic disease.
- Total iron binding capacity is increased in iron deficiency.
- Total iron binding capacity is decreased in anaemia of chronic disease.
- Serum ferritin level is low in iron defieciency.

Serum vitamin B_{12} and red cell folate

These will be low in deficiency states.

Schilling test

This is a test to assess vitamin B_{12} absorption and distinguishes between pernicious anaemia and terminal ileal malabsorption.

Faecal occult blood test

This is a simple test for blood in the faeces. The presence of blood suggests that there is a gastrointestinal source of bleeding, but the test is oversensitive.

Investigation of gastrointestinal haemorrhage

The upper and lower gastrointestinal tract should be investigated by endoscopy and radiological methods (see Chapters 3 and 6) such as:

- Oesophagogastroduodenoscopy.
- Colonoscopy.
- Barium meal.
- Barium enema.

Colposcopy and hysteroscopy

If there is suspected abnormal vaginal blood loss, the vagina and lining of the uterus should be inspected to look for carcinoma of the cervix or uterus or for causes of menorrhagia such as fibroids.

Mid-stream urine, intravenous urography, and cystoscopy

If there is any blood in the urine the urinary tract is investigated using intravenous urography and cystoscopy to look for renal carcinoma and urothelial tumours.

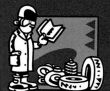

20. Postoperative Pyrexia

Many patients become pyrexial in the postoperative period and it is important that the clinician establishes the cause for this and institutes the correct treatment. The likely cause of the pyrexia is dependent not only upon the type of operation the patient has had, but also on the time after operation.

Core temperature is approximately 1°C higher than axillary temperature.

DIFFERENTIAL DIAGNOSIS OF POSTOPERATIVE PYREXIA

The differential diagnoses of the cause of pyrexia are:
- First 24 hours—trauma response, pre-existing sepsis.
- 24–72 hours postoperatively—pulmonary atelectasis, chest infection.
- 3–7 days postoperatively—chest infection, wound infection, pelvic collection or abscess, subphrenic collection or abscess, urinary tract infection, anastomotic dehiscence, wound dehiscence.
- 7–10 days postoperatively—deep venous thrombosis, pulmonary embolus.

HISTORY TO FOCUS ON THE DIFFERENTIAL DIAGNOSIS OF POSTOPERATIVE PYREXIA

Operation

It is important to know what operation has been performed. Infections are more common following large bowel procedures than following small bowel or gastric operations.

The site of operation is also important in deciding the likely source of any sepsis, for example:
- Urinary tract infection is likely following a cystoscopic procedure.
- Cholangitis is a risk in a patient who has obstructive jaundice.

Associated symptoms

Often to elicit the patient's symptoms it is necessary to ask direct questions about the following:
- Shortness of breath, productive cough, pleuritic chest pain—chest infection.
- Pain in wound, discharge—wound infection.
- Abdominal pain (worse on movement or breathing), and distension—intra-abdominal collection.
- Frequency, dysuria, haematuria, offensive urine —urinary infection.
- Calf pain, swelling of leg—deep vein thrombosis.

EXAMINATION OF PATIENTS WHO HAVE POSTOPERATIVE PYREXIA

Each system should be thoroughly examined and temperature, pulse, blood pressure, and urine output should be noted.

Features of septicaemia are rigors, high temperature, tachycardia, hypotension, and warm peripheries.

Respiratory system

On examination respiratory rate, oxygen saturation, and use of accessory muscles should be noted. The chest is examined by inspection, palpation, percussion, and auscultation.

Wound

The wound should be inspected for signs of infection including:
- Erythema—cellulitis.
- Swelling.
- Higher temperature than surrounding skin.
- Fluctuance.
- Discharge.

Abdominal examination

Following abdominal operations signs of deep infection include:

- Swinging pyrexia (see Chapter 40, Fig. 41.2) —suggesting abscess formation.
- Tenderness away from the scar.
- Peritonism—indicating local inflammation.
- Palpable swelling—due to a large collection or more frequently an inflammatory mass.
- Abdominal distension and absent bowel sounds —prolonged ileus.

Rectal examination should be performed. A pelvic abscess may be palpable as a boggy swelling through the rectal wall.

Legs

A deep vein thrombosis should be suspected if the following are present:

- Unilateral swelling of the leg.
- Increased temperature of the swollen leg compared with the other.
- Firm tender calf.

Clinical examination is, however, unreliable and further investigation should be performed (see below).

INVESTIGATION OF PATIENTS WHO HAVE POSTOPERATIVE PYREXIA

An algorithm for the investigation and diagnosis of postoperative pyrexia is given in Fig. 20.1.

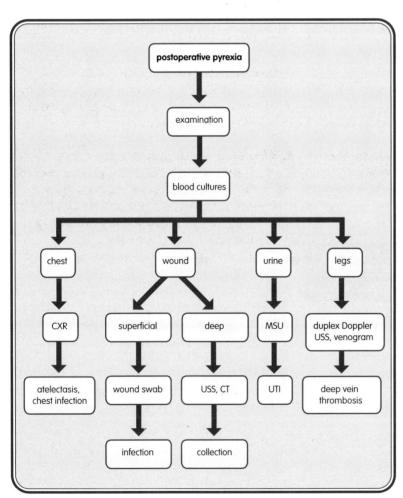

Fig. 20.1 Investigation and diagnosis of postoperative pyrexia. (CT, computed tomography; CXR, chest radiography; MSU, mid-stream urine; USS, ultrasound scan; UTI, urinary tract infection.)

Blood tests

Full blood count

This may show a high white cell count suggesting an infective cause. However, trauma of any kind (e.g. accident or surgical insult) can lead to a high white cell count. Overwhelming sepsis may cause a low white cell count.

Blood cultures

These should be requested for any pyrexial patient. The results will not be available until 48 hours later, but these can guide clinicians on the choice of antibiotics as well as give clues to the likely source of sepsis.

All culture specimens should be taken before starting antibiotics.

Chest radiography

This may show signs of:

- Collapse.
- Consolidation.
- Pleural effusion.
- Large pulmonary emboli—may show up as more lucent areas of lung (usually wedge shaped).

Electrocardiography

This is usually normal (except perhaps for a tachycardia) if there are small pulmonary emboli. If there is a large pulmonary embolus the electrocardiogram may show the following classical features:

- Tall peaked P wave in lead II—due to right atrial dilatation.
- Right axis deviation—due to right ventricular dilatation and hypertrophy.
- S1, Q3, T3 pattern—a deep S wave in I and Q wave and inverted T wave in III associated with right ventricular strain.

Arterial blood gases

In severe chest infection there may be a low pO_2 and high pCO_2. Pulmonary embolus usually results in a normal pO_2 and a low pCO_2 due to hyperventilation.

Ventilation/perfusion scanning

This is used to reveal mismatched perfusion and ventilation defects to identify pulmonary emboli.

Mid-stream urine

Urine should be sent for microscopy and culture to elucidate any infection.

Ultrasonography

An ultrasound scan is useful to look for collections, either superficial or deep. Collections can be visualized and drained under ultrasound control.

Computed tomography

Small interloop abscesses within the abdomen are often not visible on ultrasound because the gas-filled bowel loops obscure the view. Computed tomography is useful for seeing these collections and any collection in the retroperitoneal area of the abdominal cavity.

Hx from post op. patient
1. Type of op
2. Pain → specifically leg
   chest
   . ↑ing wound pain
   . Abdo pain ↑ by mvt. (collection)

3. Resp. sympts
   SOB
   haemoptysis
   productive cough
   pleuritic chest pain

3. G.I symptoms
- passage of stool/gas since op
- Any swelling of abdo?
- Appetite
- Able to eat normally
- Any N or V?

4. U.T symptoms
- Catheter?
- Passed urine since op?
- Any difficulty passing urine?
- Any pain on passing urine?

DH: Incl. analgesia
           - ABs
           - Heparin prophylaxis

Social Hx. Lives alone?
              How many stairs ...

O/E:
① Look around bed: → Drips
                          → lines
                          → drains
                          → N/g tube
                          → Urinary catheter

② Prelim. assessment:
- general impression ? - ill / pain / ↓ wt. / hydration
- MMSE ? orientated
- Hands - ? pale
- pulse
- BP
- eyes - ? sunken
- conjunctival
- sclerae - ? jaundice

③ Examine chest → ? BS ⇒ may be absent following abdo. Sx.
④ Examine abdo →
⑤ Examine wound: site/type/stiches/clips/apposition of edges/redness/swelling/bruising/discharge
⑥ Examine legs:
⑦ Examine P. areas.
⑧ Look at charts.

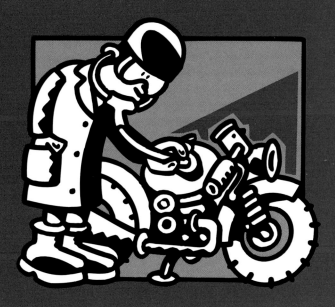

HISTORY, EXAMINATION, AND COMMON INVESTIGATIONS

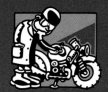

21. Clerking a Surgical Patient

INTRODUCTION

Taking an accurate and detailed history from a patient is a critical stage in making the diagnosis and provides vital information. It is important to listen and observe, let the patient tell the story in his or her own words, then use questions to clarify points. It involves acquiring information about the present problems and supplementing this with background information about related symptoms, general health, and past-medical history.

Many patients who are referred to surgeons do not need to have an operation, but require the diagnostic skills of surgeons. A surgical operation may not be the first mode of treatment, but if it is contemplated it is important that the surgeon is aware of the patient's general health and past history, which may influence:
- The type of operation that can be performed.
- The type of anaesthesia.
- The risks associated with the operation.

When clerking a surgical patient always remember to:
- Introduce yourself to the patient.
- Be polite and try to establish a rapport with the patient to help them feel at ease.
- Maintain eye contact.
- Give the patient time to express his or her thoughts.

Always remember to observe:
- The general surroundings of the patient.
- The general demeanor of the patient—anxious, in pain, comfortable, well, unwell.

Remember that the clerking of a patient is a record of your encounter with the patient and when you are qualified it is an important hospital document so it must be accurate, legible, and signed.

HISTORY

This should include the following information:
- Patient details—patient's name, age, address, marital status, occupation.

- Date, time, and place of consultation (e.g. accident and emergency department, outpatient clinic).

Presenting complaint
This is a brief statement of the reason for consulting the doctor.

History of presenting complaint
After the patient has given a brief summary of the problem it is important to obtain a more detailed history of the symptoms in a chronological order. For all the symptoms mentioned, further details are required regarding:
- Duration.
- Progression.
- Frequency.
- Severity.
- Exacerbating and relieving factors.
- Any associated symptoms.

With clinical experience vital clues from the history allow pattern recognition so the doctor can then ask more specific questions to aid the diagnostic process.

It is always important to define what the patient means by terms such as diarrhoea, constipation, or indigestion because each patient has a different experience.

Past medical history
All previous admissions to hospital, operations, any problems with anaesthesia (e.g. difficult intubation), and any unpleasant experiences (e.g. postoperative vomiting or awareness during a procedure) are documented because this will affect the patient's reaction to future operations. The patient is asked specifically about whether he or she has or has had any of the following conditions:

- Tuberculosis.
- Rheumatic fever.
- Valvular heart disease.
- Myocardial infarction.
- Cerebrovascular accident.
- Diabetes mellitus.
- Jaundice.
- Epilepsy.
- Asthma.

Systematic enquiry

Although the patient may present with a very specific problem (e.g. a hernia), it is important to assess all systems because general health and past medical history will influence the need for an operation and the type of operation that is considered appropriate (Fig 21.1).

Drug history

Ask about current medication and any recent changes of medication. Many patients cannot remember the names and dosages of their medication so gain accurate information from general practitioner records, repeat prescriptions, or labels on bottles.

Obtain information about allergic reactions and define what the patient means by an allergy—the usual symptoms are rash, oedema, difficulty breathing, but many people mention nausea and diarrhoea or 'thrush' as allergic reactions. Specific drugs that should be noted before an operation include:

- Diuretics—these decrease the potassium level and this may lead to cardiac instability.
- Insulin and diabetic medication.
- Aspirin and anticoagulants—risk of bleeding.

Fig. 21.1 Systematic enquiry.

System	Features to ask about
general	night sweats, pyrexia, jaundice, anorexia, fatigue, weight changes
cardiovascular system	chest pain, angina, exercise tolerance palpitations ankle swelling shortness of breath on exertion or lying flat, paroxysmal nocturnal dyspnoea intermittent claudication
respiratory system	cough, sputum production, haemoptysis wheezing or asthma—frequency of attacks—severity of symptoms shortness of breath, exercise tolerance
gastrointestinal system	indigestion, gastro-oesophageal reflux, dysphagia abdominal pain, vomiting, nausea bowel habit—frequency, change, difficulty rectal bleeding appetite, weight loss
genitourinary system (male)	frequency, nocturia dysuria, haematuria hesitancy, urinary stream, dribbling impotence, libido
genitourinary system (female)	menarche, menopause, pregnancies, contraception menstrual history—length of cycle, date of last menstrual period vaginal discharge dyspareunia
central nervous system	headaches, fits, faints paraesthesia, weakness dizziness, vertigo
musculoskeletal system	muscle aches, pains arthritis, poor mobility, neck stiffness

- Asthma medication—inhalers may need to be changed to nebulizers pre- and postoperatively.
- Cardiac medication and antihypertensives—should be continued.
- Anticonvulsants—should be continued.
- Corticosteroids—long-term use results in adrenal suppression and therefore corticosteroid supplements are required to cope with the stress of surgery.

Family history

Questions are asked about any illnesses that appear to occur in the family and the cause of death of first degree relatives. If a patient presents with a change of bowel habit and has a family history of colon cancer this obviously causes the patient anxiety and should also concern the doctor.

There may be a family history of anaesthetic problems (e.g. familial deficiency of pseudocholinesterase in which patients cannot metabolize short-acting muscle relaxants given during anaesthesia).

Social history

When a patient is seen in hospital it is important to remember that this is an abnormal environment where the patient feels vulnerable so obtain some more information on the patient's normal environment including:

- Occupation.
- Social circumstances—home, relatives, other people who are affected by the patient's illness.
- If elderly or dependent are social services involved?
- Financial problems that may be exacerbated by the illness.
- Smoking—average consumption and duration.
- Alcohol—average number of units per week.
- Drug abuse.
- Recent foreign travel.

INFLUENCE OF CO-EXISTING DISEASE ON OPERATIVE INTERVENTION

Approximately 50% of patients who have an operation, particularly elderly patients and those undergoing an emergency operation, have concurrent medical illnesses. Operative risks are increased in these patients, especially if they have cardiovascular or respiratory disease. Pre-operatively it is therefore important to:

- Accurately diagnose and assess medical conditions.
- Optimize medical conditions before surgery.
- Consider potential drug interactions.

IMPORTANT MEDICAL CONDITIONS

Cardiovascular conditions

The key cardiovascular conditions to consider together with the major practical points to remember for operative intervention are:

- Ischaemic heart disease—important to maintain adequate coronary artery perfusion.
- Myocardial infarction—use of a general anaesthetic within 6 months of a myocardial infarction increases the risk of a further myocardial infarction.
- Valvular heart disease—antibiotic prophylaxis is needed to prevent endocarditis.
- Mitral stenosis and atrial fibrillation—anticoagulation may be necessary.
- Severe aortic stenosis—important to maintain adequate blood pressure and coronary artery perfusion.
- Arrhythmias—stabilize preoperatively and maintain medication perioperatively.
- Hypertension—often associated with ischaemic heart disease—if diastolic blood pressure is higher than 110 mmHg it should be stabilized before surgery if possible.
- Congestive cardiac failure—if not controlled preoperatively there is a risk of further deterioration during anaesthesia.
- Pacemaker—take precautions with diathermy during surgery.

Respiratory conditions

The key conditions to consider for the respiratory system together with the major practical points to remember for operative intervention are:

- Asthma—optimize condition preoperatively.
- Chronic obstructive airways disease—if there is chronic sputum production the patient has an increased risk of respiratory infection because general anaesthesia increases the viscosity of secretions and decreases the action of the cilia. Postoperative pain may inhibit respiratory effort.
- Smoking—increased risk (× 6) of postoperative problems. It causes mucus hypersecretion, impaired

tracheobronchial clearance mechanisms, small airway narrowing, and decreased immune function. It also increases carbon monoxide concentration in the blood and decreases oxygen carrying capacity. The carbon monoxide has a negative cardiac inotropic effect and this is a risk if the patient has ischaemic heart disease. Stopping smoking 12–24 hours preoperatively has a beneficial effect on the cardiovascular system, but patients need to stop smoking 6 weeks preoperatively to gain any beneficial effect on respiratory function.

Gastrointestinal conditions

The key conditions to consider for the the gastrointestinal system together with the major practical points to remember for operative intervention are:

- Acid reflux, hiatus hernia, oesophagitis—with these conditions there is a risk of reflux at induction of anaesthesia and risk of aspiration of gastric contents into lungs. The anaesthetist will prescribe antacids and histamine H_2-receptor antagonists and apply gentle pressure to the cricoid cartilage to prevent stomach contents passing into the lungs at induction before intubation.
- Obesity—this is associated with increased morbidity and mortality rates because of the risk of cardiovascular and respiratory problems, difficult venous access, and increased risk of thromboembolic events postoperatively, and because the operation may be technically more difficult.

Endocrine conditions

The key conditions to consider for the endocrine system together with the major practical points to remember for operative intervention are as follows.

Diabetes mellitus

Operations result in impaired glucose tolerance with metabolic disturbances. Diabetics are more prone to cardiovascular problems and problems associated with autonomic neuropathy, and have an increased risk of infection.

Thyroid disorders

Local problems of a mass in the neck may result in difficult intubation. If the patient is euthyroid preoperatively and has no specific problem normal medication should be maintained.

Adrenal disorders

The problems associated with these disorders are as follows:

- Excess glucocorticoid results in problems due to increased glucose levels, increased blood pressure, and electrolyte disturbances.
- Excess mineralocorticoid results in decreased potassium levels, increased sodium levels, and hypertension.
- Insufficient mineralocorticoid results in decreased sodium levels and increased potassium levels and the patient needs intravenous hydrocortisone and close monitoring of cardiovascular status.
- Excess catecholamine causes hypertension and cardiac arrhythmias.

Blood disorders

Disorders to consider together with the major practical points to remember for operative intervention are:

- Anaemia—if chronic and haemoglobin is less than 10g/dL the patient needs transfusion (at least 48 hours preoperatively if it is to be effective).
- Haemoglobinopathy—if the patient is homozygous for sickle cell anaemia there is a risk of sickle cell crisis if hypoxia occurs during operation so the patient is kept hydrated, warm, and oxygenated.
- Haemophilia—need to give appropriate clotting factors preoperatively.

Chronic renal failure

Correct electrolytes preoperatively by dialysis. Patients have an increased risk of cardiovascular problems, anaemia, electrolyte disturbances, blood coagulation problems, and infection.

Hepatocellular disorders

These include:

- Portal hypertension, ascites, jaundice, abnormal clotting—associated with a perioperative mortality rate of more than 50%.
- Obstructive jaundice—associated with a risk of postoperative renal failure due to endotoxins from gut flora.

Alcohol and drug abuse

Particular aspects to consider include the following:

- Chronic abuse of alcohol and narcotic drugs induces hepatic enzymes so a larger dosage of anaesthetic drugs may be required to be effective.

- Problems of withdrawal due to hospital admission and operation.
- Increased risk of associated human immunodeficiency virus or hepatitis B infection, so take precautions.

Neurological disorders

Disorders to consider together with the major practical points to remember for operative intervention are:
- Epilepsy—maintain normal medication.
- Cerebrovascular accident—increased risk of progression or further cerebrovascular accident.

Rheumatoid arthritis

The anaesthetist is concerned with neck movements because of the risk of difficult intubation or subluxation if neck with an unstable atlantoaxial joint is hyperextended—so need cervical spine radiography.

COMMON PRESENTING SYMPTOMS

This section concentrates on common presenting symptoms and some specific details that should be obtained in the history.

Dysphagia (difficulty in swallowing)

Specific features that should be elicited include:
- Duration of symptoms—acute (i.e. bolus obstruction) or progressive over a few months (implies malignancy).

- Severity of symptoms—is it dry food, semisolids, fluids, or even saliva that the patient cannot swallow?
- Where does the blockage seem to be?
- A history of gastro-oesophageal reflex or hiatus hernia—may suggest a benign peptic stricture.
- Association with chest infections—for example, aspiration pneumonia.
- Sensation of 'double swallowing'—symptom of pharyngeal pouch.

Vomiting

Vomiting is an active process and involves violent contraction of the abdominal musculature forcibly expelling the gastric contents in a retrograde fashion. It is usually associated with gastrointestinal pathology, but it may be neurogenic as Ménière's disease or associated with medication. Features of vomiting are shown in Chapter 3, Fig. 3.1.

Abdominal pain

If the patient complains of abdominal pain a detailed history should be obtained regarding onset, site of pain, radiation, character, severity, duration, frequency, aggravating and relieving factors, and any associated symptoms (Fig. 21.2). Ask the patient to describe the pain in his or her own words, and they will often use descriptions such as gripping, burning, throbbing, or stabbing pain:
- Colicky pain—suggests obstruction of a hollow viscus. It is gripping in nature and fluctuates from peaks of intensity to complete relief. It is always severe and makes the patient restless.

Types of abdominal pain		
Nature	**Site**	**Possible diagnosis**
burning pain relieved by food	epigastrium	peptic ulceration
burning pain—worse on lying or bending	retrosternal	gastro-oesophageal reflux
severe constant pain relieved by leaning forward	epigastrium	pancreatic disease
increasing intensity	right hypochondrium, scapula	gall bladder disorder
sudden onset, severe, constant	generalized	peritonitis—perforated viscus
intermittent colicky	central and lower abdomen	bowel obstruction
severe colicky pain	loin, groin, scrotum	ureteric colic

Fig. 21.2 Nature, site and possible diagnosis of abdominal pain.

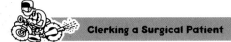

- Somatic pain—severe localized pain due to inflammation of the parietal peritoneum from localized or generalized peritonitis. It is aggravated by movement so the patient lies still.
- Burning pain—signifies mucosal injury or inflammation such as oesophagitis.

The site of the abdominal pain is related to the embryological development of the gut:
- Epigastric pain—foregut (oesophagus, stomach, duodenum).
- Central and periumbilical pain—midgut (duodenum, small intestine, right colon).
- Suprapubic pain—hindgut (mid-transverse colon, left colon, rectum).

The nature and sites of different types of abdominal pain are summarized in Fig. 21.2 with their possible diagnoses.

Change of bowel habit and rectal bleeding

If a patient complains of a change of bowel habit it is important to define the previous bowel habit (i.e. frequency and consistency of motion and colour).

Everyone has their own idea of what is 'normal'. Constipation may mean infrequent bowel action or difficulty in evacuation or hard stool. Diarrhoea may mean increased frequency and number of bowel actions or change of consistency.

Associated symptoms are:
- Passage of blood or mucus.
- Tenesmus (i.e. a sensation of incomplete evacuation of the rectum).

If there is rectal bleeding it is important to know its relationship to defaecation (i.e. is the blood mixed with faeces or separate and occurring after defaecation).
If it is:
- Bright red and fresh it is probably arising from the anal canal or low rectum.
- Dark red and mixed with the stool it is coming from the upper rectum or sigmoid colon.

Jaundice

If the presenting complaint is jaundice then associated features are colour of urine and faeces and any history of pruritus. Associated symptoms are anorexia, nausea, abdominal pain, weight loss, and pyrexia.

Clues to the aetiology may come from a history of gallstones, drug history, a history of foreign travel, and contact with infectious illnesses such as hepatitis.

Lump

If the patient complains of a lump then clarify the duration of the history:
- When did the lump appear?
- Is there any change in size or consistency?
- Is there any pain or tenderness or inflammation?
- Are there any associated symptoms such as bleeding or discharge?

If a hernia is suspected:
- Does the lump disappear spontaneously?
- Are there any precipitating factors such as chronic cough, constipation, urinary difficulties, or history of heavy lifting?
- Has there been any episode of colicky abdominal pain, vomiting, and tenderness of the lump that may suggest obstruction?

Breast problems

Breast complaints are usually of a breast lump, breast pain, or nipple discharge.

Features of a breast lump are:
- Its relationship to the menstrual cycle—has it changed in size with the cycle?
- Is there any associated discomfort?

Benign lumps often show cyclical variation.

If there is a discharge, its colour and whether it is from a single duct or many ducts are relevant.

If the complaint is of breast pain then its intensity and relationship to the menstrual cycle needs to be clarified.

A history of breast problems is not complete unless there is a record of the menstrual history including:
- Age of menarche.
- Number of pregnancies.
- Age at first pregnancy.
- Use of oral contraceptive or hormone replacement therapy.
- Any family history of breast cancer.

Thyroid disorders

Does the patient have any symptoms of hypo- or hyperthyroidism such as:
- Weight gain, lethargy, constipation, cold intolerance, dry hair—hypothyroidism.

- Weight loss, anxiety, tremor, palpitations, heat intolerance, diarrhoea—hyperthyroidism.

Are there any symptoms from compression (e.g. dysphagia, dyspnoea, hoarse voice).

Peripheral vascular disease

If the patient complains of a cramp-like pain in the calf while walking that is relieved by rest it suggests intermittent claudication (claudicare—to limp). The claudication distance reflects the severity of the symptoms. The pain is due to ischaemia and the accumulation of metabolites such as lactic acid during exertion.

Rest pain is constant severe pain in the legs that is worse at night and often made easier by sleeping in a chair. This implies critical ischaemia and may be exacerbated by infection or ulceration. Associated problems are diabetes mellitus, ischaemic heart disease, and cerebrovascular disease. There is usually a history of smoking.

Urinary symptoms

The main symptoms are:
- Dysuria (i.e. painful micturition).
- Frequency—how often the patient micturates.
- Nocturia—micturition at night.
- Urgency—poor control.
- Hesitancy with poor stream and terminal dribbling —suggest outflow obstruction.
- Haematuria—blood in the urine needs to be defined as macroscopic or microscopic.

Questions need to be asked about whether the blood is fresh or altered and whether it occurs:
- At the start of micturition—suggesting that it comes from the urethra.
- Throughout micturition—therefore possibly from the kidney or bladder.
- At the end of micturiton—comes from the prostatic bed.

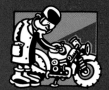

22. Examination of a Surgical Patient

Examination of any patient should be conducted in a systematic manner to ensure that nothing is missed. The extent of the 'surgical' examination does vary according to the situation—it is brief in the outpatient clinic for removal of a skin lesion, and more comprehensive if the patient is an emergency admission and has acute abdominal pain.

Examination often focuses on a specific anatomical region, but if operative intervention is contemplated the cardiovascular, respiratory, and central nervous systems should be fully assessed preoperatively.

Before touching the patient, gain an overall assessment of the patient—is the patient anxious, relaxed, in pain, well, or unwell?

EXAMINATION OF SPECIFIC SURGICAL CONDITIONS

Examination of an ulcer

An ulcer is defined as an area of discontinuity of the surface epithelium and can occur internally or externally. The basic structure and characteristic shapes of ulcers are shown in Fig. 18.1 (see p. 74).

Certain characteristics of the ulcer provide clues regarding the nature of the ulcer. Any description of the ulcer should include:
- Anatomical site.
- Floor.
- Base and edges.
- Size.
- Shape.
- Surrounding skin.
- Regional lymph nodes.

Examination of a lump or swelling

A lump may be visible on inspection, but may not be evident until palpation. The important features of a lump are:
- Anatomical site and anatomical plane (e.g. intracutaneous, subcutaneous, intramuscular).
- Size—measurements rather than comparison with objects!
- Shape, colour, temperature.

- Tenderness—if there is inflammation.
- Mobility of mass in relationship to skin and deep structures.
- Consistency—soft, hard, firm, rubbery.
- Transillumination—in darkened surroundings a light is shone through a swelling to see whether it transmits the light and therefore contains fluid.
- Fluctuation—another test for fluid, which is tested in two planes at right angles.
- Pulsations and thrills—real or transmitted.

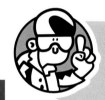

An intramuscular mass is less obvious if the muscles are contracted.

GENERAL EXAMINATION OF THE PATIENT

The following should be assessed in the general examination of the patient:
- Height and weight.
- Pulse, blood pressure, temperature.
- State of hydration—skin turgor and elasticity, sunken eyes.
- Anaemia, jaundice, cyanosis.

Common clinical signs and aetiologies

Examination of the hands (Fig. 22.1) and skin (Fig. 22.2) can reveal signs that aid in the diagnosis.

EXAMINATION OF THE BREAST

This requires removal of the clothes to the waist, a warm environment, and the presence of a chaperone. Many women will be embarrassed by the examination so be as sensitive as possible. Examination of the breast also includes examination of regional lymph nodes—axilla and supraclavicular fossa.

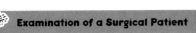

Examination of the hands	
Sign	**Diagnostic inference**
clubbing	inflammatory bowel disease, chronic lung disease, congenital heart disease
leukonychia (white patches on nails)	may be normal, liver disease
koilonychia (brittle or spoon-shaped nails)	iron deficiency anaemia
pallor of nails and palmar creases	anaemia
Dupuytren's contracture (thickening and shortening of palmar fascia causing a flexion deformity)	liver disease, epilepsy, idiopathic, familial
palmar erythema	liver disease
nicotine stains	chronic smoker
splinter haemorrhages	vasculitis, infective endocarditis
tremor and sweaty palms	thyrotoxicosis, anxiety
flap	carbon dioxide retention, hepatic encephalopathy
joint deformities	rheumatoid arthritis
Heberden's nodes of terminal interphalangeal joints	osteoarthritis

Fig. 22.1 Hand signs and their significance.

Examination of the skin	
Sign	**Diagnostic inference**
petechiae (red or blue lesions in skin deep to the epidermis)	suggests capillary fragility
spider naevi (central arterial dot from which several dilated vessels radiate)	liver disease
telangiectasia (dilatation of superficial veins)	hereditary, alcoholism, radiotherapy
cutaneous striae	previous pregnancy, weight loss, Cushing's syndrome
purpura, ecchymoses	bleeding abnormality
erythema ab igne	chronic pain
xanthelasma, arcus senilis	hyperlipidaemia
collateral veins	obstruction of normal circulation

Fig. 22.2 Skin signs and their significance.

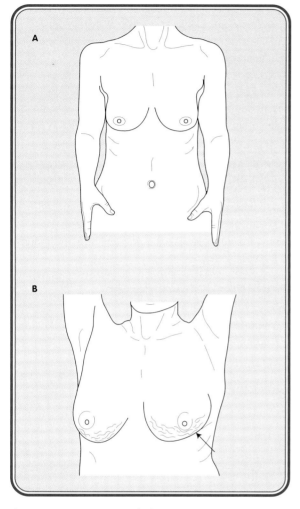

Fig. 22.3 Patient positions for breast examination. **(A)** Initial inspection is carried out with the patient sitting up with her hands by her side. **(B)** The patient is then asked to lift up her arms. This may reveal asymmetry (arrow) due to underlying disease as shown here.

Inspection of the breast

Initial inspection is done with the patient sitting up with hands by the side (Fig. 22.3A). Features to look for are:
- Any asymmetry.
- Distortion.
- Nipple abnormality.
- Redness.
- Inflammation.
- Peau d'orange of skin.

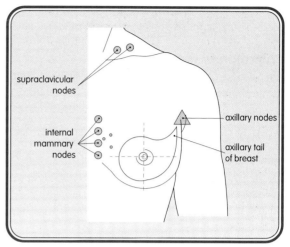

Fig. 22.4 Lymphatic drainage of the breast.

The patient then lifts her arms above her head and this accentuates any distortion or skin dimpling and allows inspection of the inframammary fold (Fig. 22.3B).

The nipple and areola are inspected for ulceration or inversion, which may be longstanding or of recent onset. Accessory nipples are very common and can occur anywhere from axilla to groin.

Palpation of the breast

The patient then lies flat or semirecumbent with her arms elevated above the head. The 'normal' breast is palpated first. If the patient is premenopausal the best time for examination is 7–10 days after a period when benign nodularity decreases. Palpation is with the flat of the fingers and is performed in a systematic fashion to incorporate all quadrants of the breast, including areola and axillary tail (Fig. 22.4). If any nipple discharge occurs its colour and whether it originates from a single or multiple ducts is noted.

If a breast lump is identified, note its characteristics of:
- Size.
- Shape.
- Position.
- Borders.
- Consistency.
- Skin tethering.

Muscle fixation is tested by asking the patient to contract pectoralis major muscle and then testing mobility.

Palpation of the axilla

The axilla is palpated when the patient is sitting upright or in a semirecumbent position. The patient's left arm is supported by the examiner's left arm so the muscles are relaxed. The examiner palpates the left axilla with his right hand and vice versa. Palpation starts at the apex of the axilla, followed by the medial (chest) wall, anterior wall, (pectoral muscles), and posterior wall (subscapularis muscle). Any nodes identified are described by:

- Number.
- Consistency.
- Mobility.

EXAMINATION OF NECK AND THYROID

Inspection of neck and thyroid

The neck is inspected from the front to look for any obvious masses such as an enlarged thyroid, lymph nodes, or salivary glands.

Dilated superficial veins may imply right ventricular failure or superior vena cava obstruction.

If the swelling is a thyroid gland it will move on swallowing because it is invested by the pretracheal fascia, which is attached to the hyoid bone.

The thyroid is bilobed with the isthmus lying over the second and third tracheal rings. The gland may be uniformly or partially enlarged.

Palpation of neck and thyroid

The thyroid gland is palpated by the examiner standing behind the patient. Palpation may demonstrate a diffusely enlarged gland or a solitary nodule. The consistency of the thyroid is either smooth, multinodular, or hard and fixed. The swelling may extend to the superior mediastinum if its inferior margin is impalpable. The trachea may be deviated by a unilateral swelling.

A midline swelling that moves when the tongue is protruded is a thyroglossal cyst.

Auscultation of a thyroid goitre may demonstrate a bruit if it is a hypervascular thyrotoxic goitre. There may be stridor if there is involvement of the recurrent laryngeal nerve or compression of trachea by a large goitre.

Examination of the thyroid is not complete without looking for signs of hypothyroidism or thyrotoxicosis and the eye changes of exophthalmos, lid lag, and ophthalmoplegia.

If palpation of the neck reveals enlarged lymph nodes their position and characteristics should be described and all anatomical areas that drain to those nodes should be examined to identify the primary lesion.

EXAMINATION OF THE ABDOMEN

The regions of the abdomen are shown in Fig. 22.5. In a warm environment the patient lies supine with one pillow. The abdomen is exposed from the xiphisternum to the pubic area.

Inspection of the abdomen

The inspection consists of noting:

- Abdominal wall movement on respiration.
- Scars, striae, ostomies.

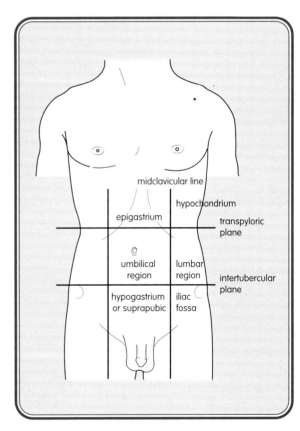

Fig. 22.5 Anatomical regions of the abdomen.

- Distension and contour of abdomen.
- Peristalsis and pulsation.
- Dilated veins and bruising.
- Erythema ab igne.

Palpation of the abdomen
The examiner should have warm hands! He or she kneels by the bed or raises the bed so that the arm is parallel to the abdomen. Palpation is carried out with the flat of the fingers. Initially it is light, then deeper and then the organs and masses are palpated.

Acute abdomen
In the acute situation the patient will be apprehensive. Palpation starts in an area that is not painful so that there is no voluntary muscle spasm to confuse the picture.

If there is any peritonitis, the peritoneum is inflamed and the overlying muscles become tense due to stimulation of the somatic nerves supplying the abdominal parietes. The pain is made worse by movement or pressure and the act of coughing or simple percussion over the affected area may produce marked pain to be diagnostic of peritonitis.

The extent of abdominal wall rigidity is affected by the state of the individual's musculature (elderly, frail patients may have minimal muscle tone despite peritonitis, but younger people have 'board-like' rigidity). Patients taking corticosteroids may not exhibit the classical signs of peritonism.

If there is diffuse peritonism deep palpation should not be carried out. If there is localized tenderness the rest of the abdomen should be examined more deeply.

Specific clinical signs include:
- Tenderness over McBurney's point (one-third of the distance between the anterior superior iliac crest and umbilicus)—suggests localized peritonism associated with appendicitis.
- Murphy's sign—localized tenderness in the right hypochondrium, accentuated while palpating the area during deep inspiration—a sign of acute cholecystitis.

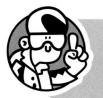
During palpation of the abdomen watch the patient's facial expression.

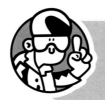
Never forget to examine hernial orifices if the patient has an acute abdomen.

Palpation of abdominal masses
Liver and gall bladder
The lower edge of the liver may be palpable normally. Palpation of the liver starts from the right iliac fossa and proceeds towards the right hypochondrium. The patient breathes in and out as the examiner's hand moves.
If a liver edge is found then its characteristics are noted. It may be:
- Smooth.
- Craggy.
- Tender.
- Enlarged (note the degree of enlargement).

A normal gall bladder is not palpable, but if it is distended it may be a round smooth swelling palpable at the liver edge in the midclavicular line.

Spleen
The spleen lies beneath the left ninth, tenth, and eleventh ribs on the abdomen's posterolateral wall. It has to be enlarged by 1.5–2 times normal before it is palpable. It enlarges medially and inferiorly so it projects below the costal margin towards the right iliac fossa. There is a notch on its medial aspect. Palpation therefore starts from right iliac fossa and moves towards the left hypochondrium.

Kidneys
Normal kidneys are not palpable, but an enlarged kidney may be palpable as a mass in the loin, which moves on respiration and is ballotable when examined bimanually (i.e. one hand anteriorly and one posteriorly).
The characteristics and anatomical position of any abdominal mass will give vital clues to its aetiology (Fig. 5.1, p. 21).

Percussion of the abdomen
This is useful if the abdomen is distended. A resonant note suggests gaseous distension of a viscus. If the note is resonant centrally and becomes dull in the flanks there may be fluid present. This can be confirmed by examining the patient when he or she is lying on one

side and the dullness then shifts. A fluid thrill may also be present if there is ascites.

Causes of abdominal distension are flatus, fluid, fat, foetus, or faeces.

Auscultation of the abdomen

The stethoscope is used to listen for bowel sounds, which may be:

- Absent despite listening for 2 min—suggests an adynamic ileus.
- Hyperactive—imply increased peristaltic activity.
- High-pitched and tinkling—occur when fluid is moving around in a distended obstructed loop of intestine.

A succussion splash occurs when the stomach is obstructed and full of fluid and it is heard when the patient is moved from side to side.

Bruits may be heard over narrowed arteries.

Rectal examination

Examination of the abdomen is not complete without a rectal examination. Women who have acute abdominal pain should also have a vaginal examination. The rectum is examined with the patient in the left lateral position with knees flexed. The perianal region is inspected for:

- Signs of inflammation.
- Fistula.
- Fissures.
- Skin tags.
- Prolapsed haemorrhoids.

A lubricated finger is then gently inserted, but in the presence of acute problems this may be too uncomfortable. If possible the tone of the anal sphincter is assessed. Each wall of the rectum is palpated for local tenderness, inflammation, and mucosal lesions, and the size and consistency of the prostate is noted. In the acute situation deep tenderness may be associated with:

- Acute appendicitis.
- Salpingitis.
- Prostatitis.

A ballooned rectum may be found in a patient who has pseudo-obstruction.

EXAMINATION OF A HERNIA

If a groin hernia is suspected, the patient should be examined standing up because it may reduce when the patient lies down. Observe the position of the swelling—if it descends towards the scrotum this is likely to be an indirect inguinal hernia. Palpation over the swelling as the patient coughs produces a cough impulse.

The patient then lies down. If the swelling disappears immediately it is a direct inguinal hernia. If the swelling has to be reduced, but is controlled by pressure over the deep inguinal ring (halfway between the pubic symphysis and the anterior superior iliac spine) it is an indirect inguinal hernia.

A femoral hernia is most commonly seen in women and is found below the inguinal ligament; the neck is below and lateral to the pubic tubercle.

If a hernia is inflamed, tender, and irreducible then it is probably acutely obstructed and the contents are at risk of strangulation.

Other hernias may be visible when the patient is standing, but not when the patient is lying. They may be visible by asking the patient to cough or lift their legs or head off the bed by contracting the rectus abdominis muscles.

EXAMINATION OF A SCROTAL SWELLING

Patients can be examined lying or standing. If there is a scrotal swelling the first step is to see whether it is possible to get above the swelling; if it is not the swelling is an inguinoscrotal hernia.

If the swelling is a scrotal swelling:

- Is it uni- or bilateral and does the swelling transilluminate?
- Can the testis be felt separately and does it feel normal in size, shape, and lie?
- Are there any signs of inflammation?

Descriptions of scrotal swelling and their diagnoses can be seen in Fig. 22.6.

Scrotal swellings	
Description	**Diagnosis**
painless swelling of testis	testicular tumour
horizontal lie of testis, painful	testicular torsion
cystic swelling separate from testis	epididymal cyst
transilluminable swelling of scrotum, testis impalpable	hydrocele
tender epididymis	epididymitis
distended veins—'bag of worms'	varicocele

Fig. 22.6 Scrotal swellings and their significance.

EXAMINATION OF PERIPHERAL VASCULATURE

Inspection of peripheral vasculature

General inspection of the limbs may show the effects of ischaemia such as pallor, hair loss, inflammation, and gangrene. If the patient is hanging the leg over the edge of the bed then it may imply rest pain.

Palpation of peripheral vasculature

Gentle palpation will reveal temperature differences and gentle pressure on the nailbeds will indicate the speed of capillary return. All of the peripheral pulses are palpated and the character of the pulsation is noted. The limb is examined for areas of paraesthesia.

Auscultation may demonstrate bruits over narrowed vessels.

A diagram of anatomical positions of peripheral pulses is shown in Fig. 22.7

Buerger's test

The patient lies down and both legs are lifted keeping the knees straight. The legs are supported by the examiner while the patient flexes and extends the ankles and toes to the point of fatigue. If the blood supply is defective the sole of the foot becomes pale and the veins are guttered. The feet are lowered and the patient adopts a sitting position. In 2–3 min a cyanotic hue spreads over the affected foot. This sequence signifies that a major limb artery is occluded.

EXAMINATION OF VARICOSE VEINS

Fig. 22.8 shows a diagram of normal venous drainage of the leg.

Inspection of varicose veins

With the patient standing and in good light the legs are inspected from the front and behind to assess the anatomical distribution of the varicosities affecting the long and short saphenous veins and their effects on the tissues such as hyperpigmentation, varicose excema, venous flares, oedema, lipodermatosclerosis, and ulceration. The groin is inspected to look for a saphena varix.

Palpation of varicose veins

Sometimes the veins are not obvious on inspection, but are palpable.

Tests that can be carried out when palpating veins include:
• Cough impulse.
• Trendelenburg's test.
• Percussion.

With the cough impulse test, fingers are placed over the long saphenous vein just below the

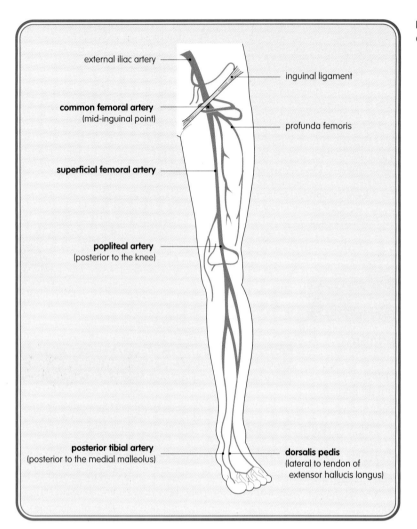

Fig. 22.7 Anatomical positions of peripheral pulses.

saphenous opening, the patient coughs and there is a palpable fluid thrill if the saphenofemoral junction is incompetent.

In the percussion test, the examiner's left fingers are placed below the saphenous opening and the other hand taps the varicosities. If the valves are incompetent then the impulse will be transmitted up the vein to the saphenous opening.

During Trendelenburg's test, the patient lies on the couch and the leg is elevated to drain the blood from the veins. Fingers are placed firmly over the saphenous opening or a tourniquet is placed around the leg. Maintaining the pressure the limb is lowered and the patient stands. If the varicose veins have been controlled

then the main incompetence is at the saphenofemoral junction. If there is partial filling of the lower varicose veins it implies that some of the lower perforating veins are also incompetent.

EXAMINATION OF A PATIENT WHO HAS MULTIPLE INJURIES

Trauma is the leading cause of death in the first four decades of life. The quality of the initial assessment has a significant influence on the final outcome. Principles of trauma management have now been well defined to improve standards of care.

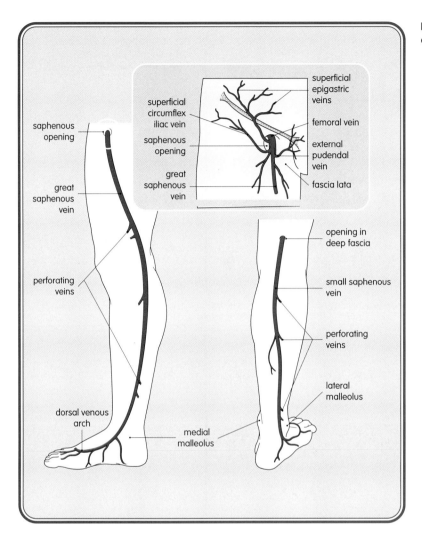

Fig. 22.8 Normal venous drainage of the leg.

Patient management consists of:
- Primary survey.
- Resuscitation.
- Secondary survey.

The aim is to detect the life-threatening injuries first and to prevent further damage to vital organs from hypoxia and hypovolaemia (Fig. 22.9). The secondary survey then looks for the non-life-threatening injuries that may have significant long-term effects if not treated properly.

Any unconscious patient should be assessed carefully with particular attention to maintaining a patent airway, blood pressure, pulse, and adequate respiration. The conscious level is assessed using the Glasgow Coma Scale (Fig. 22.10) by monitoring three features that change with the conscious level:
- Stimulus needed to cause eye opening.
- Verbal response.
- Best motor response.

The Glasgow Coma Scale is a reproducible scale so any change in level can be detected and communicated easily. A fully conscious person has a score of 15 while the deepest level of coma scores 3. A score of 8 or less indicates coma.

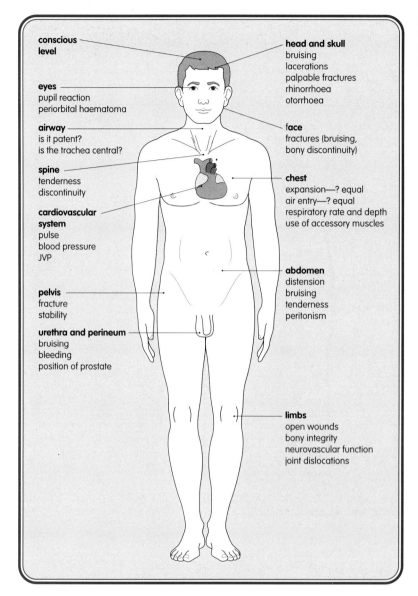

conscious level

eyes
pupil reaction
periorbital haematoma

airway
is it patent?
is the trachea central?

spine
tenderness
discontinuity

cardiovascular system
pulse
blood pressure
JVP

pelvis
fracture
stability

urethra and perineum
bruising
bleeding
position of prostate

head and skull
bruising
lacerations
palpable fractures
rhinorrhoea
otorrhoea

face
fractures (bruising,
bony discontinuity)

chest
expansion—? equal
air entry—? equal
respiratory rate and depth
use of accessory muscles

abdomen
distension
bruising
tenderness
peritonism

limbs
open wounds
bony integrity
neurovascular function
joint dislocations

Fig. 22.9 Areas to be examined carefully in patients who have suffered multiple trauma. (JVP, jugular venous pressure.)

Fig. 22.10 Glasgow Coma Scale.

Glasgow coma scale					
Eye opening		**Voice response**		**Best motor response**	
				obeys commands	6
		alert and orientated	5	localizes pain	5
spontaneous	4	confused	4	flexes to pain	4
to voice	3	inappropriate	3	abnormal flexion to pain	3
to pain	2	incomprehensible	2	extends to pain	2
no eye opening	1	no voice response	1	no response to pain	1

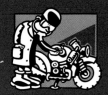
SAMPLE CLERKING

A sample surgical clerking is shown below. Abbreviations used in this sample medical clerking are GP, general practitioner; PC, presenting complaint; HPC, history of presenting complaint; PMH, past medical history; TIA, transient ischaemic attack; TB, tuberculosis; DH, drug history; od, once daily; bd, twice daily; CVS, cardiovascular system; RS, respiratory system; GI, gastrointestinal system; GU, genitourinary system; CNS, central nervous system; LS, locomotor system; FH, family history; SH, social history; JVP, jugular venous pressure; Ht sounds, heart sounds; I, first heart sound; II, second heart sound; Resp. rate, respiratory rate; R, right; L, left; HO, hernial orifices; PR, rectal examination; NAD, nothing abnormal detected; U&Es, urea and electrolytes; ECG, electrocardiogram.

DETAILS

Name:	Freda Smith
Address:	6 Town Road, London.
Date:	1st January 2000
Time:	20.30 h
Place:	Admissions Unit—referred by GP
Age:	72 years
Sex:	female
Occupation:	housewife, retired sewing machinist

PC

Acute onset of abdominal pain at 2 pm.

HPC

Sudden onset of upper abdominal pain at 2 pm, about 1 hour after lunch of fried fish.
Constant severe pain, radiates to back, exacerbated by movement.
Not relieved by antacids.
Associated symptoms—vomited bile-stained fluid several times.
Recent problems with 'indigestion', relieved by antacids. Some fatty food intolerance.
No bowel problems.
No history of jaundice.

PMH

Appendicectomy—age 10 years.
Hysterectomy—age 45 years.
TIA—6 months ago.
No TB/rheumatic fever/diabetes/epilepsy/asthma/myocardial infarction/ ↑ blood pressure.

DH

Bendrofluazide 5 mg od.
Brufen 400 mg bd.
Aspirin 75 mg od.
No known allergies.

Systematic enquiry

CVS

No chest pain/palpitations/orthopnoea/intermittent claudication.
Mild ankle oedema.

RS

No cough/sputum/haemoptysis/wheeze.
Slight shortness of breath on exertion up hills.

GI

See above

GU

No dysuria/haematuria.
Occasional frequency and urgency.
Menopause aged 50 years.

CNS

No headaches/fits/faints/paraesthesia.
Full recovery after TIA.

LS

Arthritis affecting hips and lower back.

FH

Father died of heart attack aged 73 years.
Mother died of 'old age' at 83 years.
No family history of any illnesses.

SH

Widowed—lives alone—in a first floor flat.
Non-smoker/occasional glass of sherry.
No social services.

On examination

Unwell
In pain—lying still
Temp. 37.5°C
? slightly jaundiced
No anaemia/cyanosis/clubbing/lymphadenopathy

CVS

Pulse 110/min, regular, small volume
Blood pressure 110/70 mmHg
JVP not elevated
Ht sounds I + II + nil added
Peripheral pulses palpable
slight ankle oedema

RS

Resp. rate 20/min—shallow
Trachea central
Expansion R = L
Air entry R = L
Breath sounds vesicular with scattered rhonchi

AS

Decreased abdominal movement
Diffuse tenderness and peritonism in the upper abdomen
No liver/spleen/kidneys palpable
Decreased bowel sounds
HO intact
Femoral pulses palpable
PR—NAD

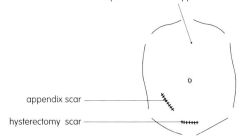

diffuse tenderness and peritonism in the upper abdomen

appendix scar

hysterectomy scar

CNS

Alert and orientated

Cranial nerves intact

Tone, power, and sensation R=L, normal

Reflexes R=L

Impression

A 72-year-old lady with a history of sudden onset of severe epigastric pain that is associated with nausea and vomiting. Mrs Smith has a previous history of indigestion and fatty food intolerance.

Differential diagnosis

Pancreatitis

Acute cholecystitis

Perforated peptic ulcer

Investigations

Blood tests—full blood count, U&Es, liver function tests, glucose, and amylase to diagnose pancreatitis

ECG to exclude myocardial infarction

Erect chest X-ray to diagnose perforation

Management

Analgesia

Investigations

Intravenous fluids

Monitoring of pulse, blood pressure, urine output, and oxygen saturation

Further management depends upon the results of investigations

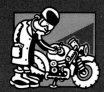

24. Investigation of a Surgical Patient

After clerking the patient, a list of differential diagnoses is formulated. This will aid the selective planning of further investigations. When planning further investigations, it is important to remember:

- If the patient is an acute admission, there is a limit to the investigations that can be requested in the middle of the night.
- Do not order a long list of investigations hoping that one will provide the answer.
- Students should try and see as many investigations being carried out as possible so that they are aware of the nature of the tests and what the patients have to experience.
- Some tests are very straightforward, but others require specialists to perform them.

ASSESSMENT BEFORE GENERAL ANAESTHESIA

Young fit patients may require no investigations before a minor elective operation, but any patient who has a history of respiratory or cardiovascular problems needs to be assessed by:

- Electrocardiogram (ECG)—to detect arrhythmias, ischaemic changes, previous myocardial infarction and evidence of hypertrophy. This is not required if the patient is under 40 years of age, asymptomatic, and has no risk factors.
- Chest radiograph—incidence of abnormalities is 10% in patients over 40 and 25% in patients over 60 years of age, respectively. A chest radiograph is not required if the patient is asymptomatic, has no risk factors, and is under 50 years of age. A chest radiograph can shows signs of chronic lung disease, cardiomegaly, and signs of cardiac failure.

Specialized tests of respiratory and cardiovascular function
These are:

- Echocardiography—to assess valvular heart disease and ventricular function.

- Exercise ECG—to diagnose angina and assess severity.
- 24-hour ECG—if the patient has a history of intermittent arrhythmias.
- Peak expiratory flow rate—to assess asthma.
- Lung function tests—to measure forced expiratory volume in 1 s and forced vital capacity to assess lung function of patients who have chronic lung disease.
- Blood gas analysis—arterial blood sample is analysed for oxygen and carbon dioxide levels. If these are abnormal they may indicate the possibility of postoperative chest problems.

Blood tests
Full blood count
Measurements include:

- Haemoglobin level—decreased in anaemia, increased in polycythaemia and dehydration.
- Mean corpuscular haemoglobin and mean corpuscular volume—decreased in iron deficiency anaemia.
- Mean corpuscular haemoglobin—increased in vitamin B_{12} or folate deficiency or alcoholism.
- White cell count—increased if there is infection. Neutrophilia results from bacterial infection, lymphocytosis from viral infection, and eosinophilia from allergy. White cell count is decreased in overwhelming infection.
- Platelets—increased if there has been recent haemorrhage, after splenectomy, or in myeloproliferative disorders. Platelets are decreased if there is hypersplenism or in some autoimmune conditions (e.g. idiopathic thrombocytopenic purpura).

Urea and electrolytes
It is important to know the patient's preoperative renal function, especially if the patient is to have an emergency or major operation. Increased urea and creatinine may be due to dehydration or renal impairment. It is also important to know the potassium levels because if less than 3 mmol/L

the patient has an increased risk of developing cardiac arrhythmias.

Glucose

A random sample may reveal undiagnosed diabetes mellitus, particularly in the elderly. If the patient is known to be diabetic then the glucose needs to be stabilized preoperatively.

Blood transfusion

Many elective operations do not require a blood transfusion, but the patient's blood is grouped and the serum saved in case it is needed. Blood donations are now separated into a large number of different components so they can be used specifically. Whole blood is only given for acute haemorrhage; other components of blood are used as follows.

- Packed cells—given for symptomatic anaemia or urgent operation. Platelet concentrates have to be ABO/Rhesus compatible and are given if the platelet count less than 40×10^9/L.
- Clotting factors—can be infused as fresh frozen plasma and are used if there is bleeding, massive transfusion, or disseminated intravascular coagulation (DIC).
- Specific clotting factors—these are cryoprecipitate (factor VIII, von Willebrand's factor, and fibrinogen) and factor VIII and factor IX concentrates.

Adverse effects of transfusion are:
- Pyrogenic febrile reaction.
- Hypersensitivity reaction to platelet and leucocyte antigens—causes a mild pyrexia.
- Anaphylactoid reaction—may cause hypotension and bronchospasm.
- Acute haemolytic reaction—due to ABO incompatability. The clinical features are pain at the infusion site, chest pain, fever, rigors, hypotension, flushing, DIC, and renal failure. Treatment is to stop the transfusion and treat the symptoms; the patient may need dialysis.
- Metabolic haemostatic complications of a massive rapid transfusion—hypothermia, acidosis, and lack of clotting factors.
- Transmission of infectious diseases such as hepatitis C—occurs in less than 0.1% of transfusions. Blood donations in the UK are screened for hepatitis B and human immunodeficiency virus infection.

No medical or surgical condition justifies a transfusion of less than 2 units.

Specialist blood tests

You should be aware of the following specialist blood tests:
- Clotting screen—this includes the platelet count, prothrombin time, and thromboplastin time. This is performed if the patient is anticoagulated or jaundiced, or has a hepatic disorder or history of excessive bleeding.
- Sickle cell test—should be performed on all patients who come from the Middle East, Indian subcontinent, Africa, or Mediterranean areas.
- Liver function tests—these include bilirubin, hepatic transaminases, albumin, alkaline phosphatase, and γ-glutamyl transferase. Increased bilirubin and very high transaminases suggest hepatitis, but increased bilirubin and alkaline phosphatase suggest biliary obstruction or hepatic metastases.
- Hepatitis screen—if jaundiced or past history of hepatitis because the patient may be an asymptomatic carrier.
- Amylase—measured in all cases of acute abdominal pain because if it is higher than 1000 IU/L it is diagnostic of acute pancreatitis, but it can also be elevated in renal impairment or if the patient has a perforated viscus or ischaemic bowel.
- Erythrocyte sedimentation rate and C-reactive protein (an acute phase protein)—elevated in inflammatory conditions, infection, and tissue injury.

Tumour markers

These are substances present in the body in a concentration that is related to the presence of a tumour, but they may not be tumour specific (Fig. 24.1). They can be used to monitor response to treatment and early diagnosis of recurrence.

Microbiological tests

If any infection is suspected, specimens should be taken before starting antibiotics so that they can be examined microscopically and cultured to detect the organisms and their sensitivities (M, C, & S).

Fig. 24.1 Tumour markers.

Tumour markers	
Marker	Tumour
human chorionic gonadotrophin (HCG), α-fetoprotein (AFP)	testicular tumours
carcinoembryonic antigen (CEA)	colon cancer
CA125	ovarian cancer
prostatic-specific antigen (PSA)	prostatic cancer
AFP	hepatocellular carcinoma
C19–9	pancreatic cancer

Fig. 24.2 Classification of preoperative state—American Society of Anesthesiologists criteria.

Classification of preoperative state—American Society of Anesthesiologists criteria	
Class	Definition
1	healthy patient
2	mild systemic disease; no functional limitations
3	severe systemic disease with functional limitation
4	severe systemic disease that is a constant threat to life
5	moribund patient not expected to survive 24 hours with or without operation

- Pus swabs—can be taken from a wound, ulcer, or abscess.
- Mid-stream urine (MSU)—if urinary tract infection suspected. A pure culture of more than 10^5 organisms/mL is diagnostic.
- Blood cultures—these should be taken (using a sterile technique) from any patient who has a rigor or temperature of 39°C, which are signs of bacteraemia.

Classification of preoperative state

The criteria defined by the American Society of Anesthesiologists for classification of the preoperative state are given in Fig. 24.2.

INVESTIGATION OF THE GASTROINTESTINAL TRACT

Plain radiography

In the acute situation an erect chest radiograph and an abdominal radiograph are helpful. A chest radiograph will demonstrate gas under the diaphragm (Fig. 24.3). Its presence indicates a perforated viscus, but its absence does not exclude the diagnosis.

An abdominal radiograph can demonstrate several structures:

- Small bowel dilatation (Fig. 24.4)—central loops of bowel with complete lines due to the plicae circulares. It is abnormal if the small bowel is dilated.
- Colonic dilatation—this is recognized by the peripheral position of the colon and incomplete lines across the bowel due to the haustra. It can be normal.
- Gas in the biliary tree—may be due to a fistula from the gall bladder to the duodenum, which may present as a gall stone ileus.
- Loss of psoas shadow—due to retroperitoneal pathology.
- Calcification—a feature of 90% of renal tract calculi and 10% of gallstones.
- Vascular calcification—of an aneurysm and atheromatous vessels.

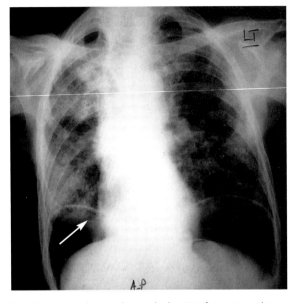

Fig. 24.3 Erect chest radiograph showing free gas under the diaphragm (arrow) and a chest infection..

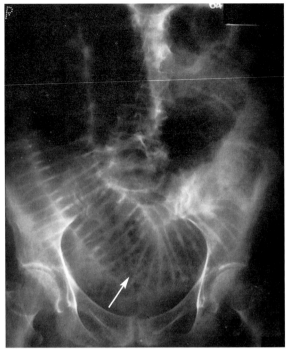

Fig. 24.4 Abdominal radiograph demonstrating small bowel dilatation (arrow).

Contrast studies

These can provide an assessment of diseases of hollow organs. Double contrast means that barium is given initially and then the viscus is distended with air and this demonstrates mucosal detail. These investigations include:

- Barium swallow—initial investigation for dysphagia because it can assess the position and length of a stricture or define the anatomy of a hiatus hernia. It is also a dynamic test for observing oesophageal motility.
- Barium meal—useful for assessing the stomach and duodenum if endoscopy is impossible (Fig. 24.5).
- Barium meal and follow-through—a nasogastric tube is passed into the stomach and barium is passed down it and then it moves into the small intestine. Radiographs are taken over a period of a few hours to monitor the progress of the barium. It is useful for assessing small bowel diseases such as Crohn's disease.
- Barium enema—a single contrast study can be performed on unprepared bowel if colonic obstruction suspected. A double contrast study can be used to assess mucosal problems after the use of aperients to clear the colon.

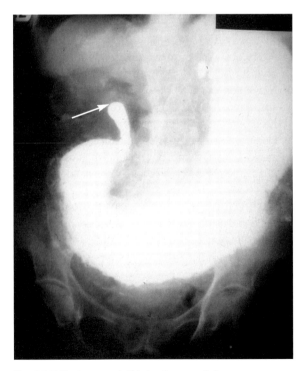

Fig. 24.5 Barium meal. This barium meal shows gross gastric distension due to pyloric obstruction (arrow).

Ultrasonography

This is a diagnostic technique that uses high-frequency sound waves to generate an image. The interfaces of different body tissues reflect the sound waves as echoes, which are converted into electrical impulses and then into images. It is very useful for examination of the biliary and urogenital systems because the contrast between fluid-filled organs, normal tissues, and calculi can lead to variations in echogenicity.

Ultrasonography is a painless investigation, but is operator dependent.

Practical aspects of note when using ultrasound for investigating different parts of the body include the following:

- Abdominal ultrasound—patients are starved for a few hours before the test to decrease bowel gas. The procedure is useful for assessing the liver, gall bladder, biliary tree, pancreas, aneurysms, inflammatory masses, and kidneys.
- Pelvic ultrasound—the patient's bladder should be full because this provides a better contrast background than air-filled bowel. This is useful for assessing gynaecological pathology and pregnancy.
- Intraluminal ultrasound—ultrasound probes can be passed down the oesophagus to assess the extent of oesophageal tumours and through the anal canal to assess rectal tumours or the anal sphincters.
- Intraoperative ultrasound—at laparotomy probes can be used to identify intrahepatic and small pancreatic tumours such as insulinoma.

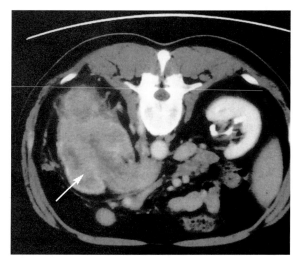

Fig. 24.6 Computed tomography scan showing renal carcinoma (arrow).

- Interventional ultrasound—biopsies and cytopathology can be taken from intra-abdominal masses using ultrasound guidance. Fluid collections can be aspirated and hydronephrotic kidneys can be drained.

Computed tomography

Computed tomography (CT) is a technique that produces cross-sectional images of the body. The CT scanner takes many images in different directions and these are fed into a digital computer, which constructs the cross-sectional image The system is very sensitive so differences in tissue density can be recognized and a detailed two-dimensional image is formed. A CT scan shows renal carcinoma in Fig. 24.6.

Magnetic resonance imaging

Magnetic resonance imaging (MRI) is a newer diagnostic tool based on the fact that an externally applied magnetic field causes protons in tissues to align in the direction of the magnetic field. By applying a second smaller magnetic field, in the form of a radiofrequency pulse, perpendicular to the main magnetic field the alignment of the protons is changed. When the radiofrequency pulse is stopped the protons return to the equilibrium and in doing this they produce another radiofrequency signal. This signal is the MR signal, which is amplified and transformed by the computer into an image.

Magnetic resonance imaging is particularly useful for imaging the central nervous system, but it also produces very high quality images of the rest of the body. The differences between vessels, tumour, inflammatory lesions and surgical scars is more easily demonstrated with MRI scans than CT scans. The presence of any metal, however, produces a marked artefact.

Radionuclide imaging

Radionuclide imaging techniques use radioisotopes to depict function rather than anatomy. The principle is that an inhaled, injected, or ingested pharmaceutical compound labelled with a suitable radionuclide is concentrated in the organ under review and the emitted radiation is detected by a gamma camera. Using the appropriate isotopes the technique can be used to look at the brain, bones, thyroid, kidney, bowel, and liver.

Radiolabelled red cells can be used to investigate bleeding from the gastrointestinal tract. If a Meckel's diverticulum is suspected technetium pertechnetate can be used to look for ectopic gastric mucosa.

Technetium-iminodiacetic acid derivatives (HIDA) can be used to investigate hepatobiliary function. These derivatives are taken up by the hepatocytes and excreted in the bile, with accumulation in the gall bladder and small intestine. This technique can be used to investigate cholecystitis and cholestasis, detect bile leakage, and assessment after hepatic transplantation.

Endoscopic techniques

The development of fibreoptic endoscopes and video viewing has revolutionized the diagnosis and management of gastrointestinal pathology. Diagnostic biopsies, excision of polyps, injection of sclerosants, insertion of stents, and removal of stones can be carried out via the endoscope. Most of the examinations are performed under sedation although most people can tolerate a diagnostic gastroscopy after local anaesthesia to the pharynx only. The examinations include:

- Oesophagogastroduodenoscopy (OGD)—examines the oesophagus, stomach, and first two parts of duodenum.
- Endoscopic retrograde cholangiopancreatography (ERCP)—a side viewing scope, which views the duodenum and allows contrast to be injected into the biliary tree, extraction of gallstones, biopsies of pancreatic lesions, and insertion of stents.
- Sigmoidoscopy—a rigid scope used in the outpatient clinic to examine the rectum and distal sigmoid colon. A flexible scope will reach the splenic flexure of the colon.
- Proctoscope—a small rigid instrument to examine the anal canal.
- Colonoscopy—a flexible instrument that can examine the colon from the rectum to the caecum. Biopsies can be taken and polyps snared and retrieved.

Intraoesophageal pH monitoring and manometry

Probes are passed via the nose into the oesophagus to monitor the pH and measure the sphincter pressures. Similar probes can be used in the anal canal to measure sphincter pressures.

Percutaneous transhepatic cholangiography

In a case of obstructive jaundice with a dilated biliary tree it may not be possible to gain access with ERCP, but contrast can be injected through the skin and liver into a dilated biliary tree to outline the biliary tree and if necessary a stent can be passed via the same route to bypass the obstruction.

INVESTIGATION OF BREAST PROBLEMS

Several investigations are used to investigate breast pathology:

- Mammograms (Fig. 24.7)—these are low-dose radiographs used to image the breast. They are not used routinely for women under 35 years of age because of their lack of sensitivity in dense glandular breasts. The technique can demonstrate mass lesions, spiculated lesions, and microcalcification that can be benign or malignant.
- Ultrasound—this is useful (particularly in young women) for distinguishing between solid and cystic lesions. It can be used to perform image-guided biopsies of impalpable lesions.
- Fine-needle aspiration cytology (FNAC)—a 21-guage needle can be used to aspirate cysts or obtain cells from solid lesions. Cytopathologists can distinguish between benign and malignant cells.
- Trucut biopsy—after local anaesthetic a core biopsy can be taken to obtain a precise pathological diagnosis.

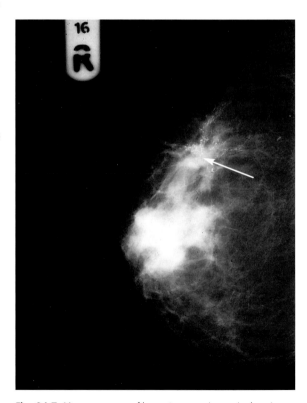

Fig. 24.7 Mammogram of breast cancer (arrow), showing a spiculated lesion with malignant microcalcification.

INVESTIGATION OF THYROID DISEASE

The following investigations can be used to test for thyroid disease:

- Thyroid function tests—thyroxine (T_4), tri-iodothyronine (T_3), and thyroid stimulating hormone (TSH). An elevated T_4 suggests thyrotoxicosis. A low T_3 and a high TSH indicate hypothyroidism.
- Thyroid antibodies—these give an indication of autoimmune disease. Antithyroglobulin and antimitochondrial antibodies are elevated in Hashimoto's disease. Long-acting thyroid stimulating antibody (LATS) is diagnostic of Graves' disease.
- Ultrasound scan—provides a simple outline of the shape of the thyroid gland and can distinguish whether a lump is solid or cystic.
- Thoracic inlet view or a chest radiograph will demonstrate tracheal displacement if compressed by a retrosternal goitre.
- Radioisotope scan—technetium pertechnetate can be used to assess thyroid function. Generalized high activity suggests Graves' disease. A highly active nodule suggests a toxic nodule and a cold nodule may indicate a tumour.
- FNAC—this can be a useful technique for diagnosing solid cold nodules suggestive of thyroid cancer.

VASCULAR INVESTIGATIONS

Vascular investigation techniques include:
- Doppler ultrasound.
- Duplex scanner.
- Ankle/brachial pressure index.
- Arteriography.
- Digital subtraction arteriography (DSA).

With Doppler ultrasound, probes can be used to detect arterial and venous blood flow. The Doppler effect is a change in frequency of a sound due to the relative movement of the source of the sound and the observer. The duplex scanner method is a pulsed Doppler combined with real time ultrasound screening, and a computer-generated picture can be used to assess flow and anatomy in the peripheral vessels, especially the carotid artery.

To measure the ankle/brachial pressure index, a Doppler probe can be used to locate the posterior tibial arterial signal. A proximally placed sphygmomanometer cuff is inflated to find the pressure at which the signal disappears and reappears on deflation. The mean of the pressures can be compared with the pressure in the arm (i.e. systemic pressure):

Ankle/brachial pressure index (ABI)
= ankle pressure/brachial pressure (%)

The ankle/brachial pressure index gives an indication of the severity of any reduction in flow and can be used as a non-invasive monitoring tool.

The retrograde (Seldinger) transfemoral arteriogram is the standard imaging technique for defining the precise abnormalities of the peripheral vascular system. The catheter is passed into the unaffected side and passed up the iliac vessels and down the affected side. Contrast medium is injected to outline the vascular system and define the level and extent of any narrowing and any collateral circulation. This can be combined with angioplasty (i.e. balloon dilatation of the vessel if there is a short segment of atherosclerosis). The risks associated with these procedures are:
- Haematoma formation.
- Initiation of intimal dissection.
- Dislodgement of thrombus.
- False aneurysm formation at the site of catheter insertion.

Digital subtraction arteriography is a new technique that is superseding the need for translumbar aortograms or arteriograms via the brachial route if both femoral vessels are included. The dye is injected into a peripheral vein and the pictures obtained are almost as good as those of conventional arteriograms, but dilutional problems result in inferior pictures of the distal vascular tree. DSA 'subtracts' the bony image and enhances the arteriographic profile.

UROLOGICAL INVESTIGATIONS

The tests to be considered in urological investigations include:
- Blood tests.
- Mid-stream urine.

Blood tests

Measurement of blood urea and creatinine levels indicate renal function and a creatinine clearance provides an estimation of the glomerular filtration rate.

Calcium, uric acid and phosphates are measured if there is stone disease.

Prostatic-specific antigen is a tumour marker for prostatic cancer.

Mid-stream urine

A ward dipstick can demonstrate the presence of glucose, ketones, blood, bilirubin, and protein, and pH.

Microscopic examination will reveal the presence of red cells, white blood cells, casts, crystals, and organisms.

A culture showing more than 10^5 bacteria/mL of a pure growth is diagnostic of a urinary tract infection.

More than three red blood cells per high power field is abnormal and more than five white cells per high power field suggests pyuria; if this is sterile it may be due to tuberculosis.

Imaging of renal tract

The different methods of imaging for the renal tract are:

- Abdominal radiograph, kidneys, ureters, and bladder (KUB view)—this may show renal calculi, renal size, or abnormal calcification (e.g. phleboliths, calcified gall stones, calcified vessels).
- Ultrasound—this is a non-invasive test that can be used to delineate the kidneys, show any evidence of obstruction (i.e. hydronephrosis) or the presence of solid or cystic lesions, measure postmicturition residual volume and assess prostate size. It can also be used to guide percutaneous renal biopsies or nephrostomy tubes. Transrectal ultrasound can be used to assess the prostate and prostatic biopsies can be obtained transrectally.
- Intravenous urography (IVU)—contrast medium (iodine based) is injected intravenously and is rapidly excreted by the kidneys if they are functioning normally. The investigation delineates the kidney and the pelvicalyceal system and it can show abnormal anatomy such as a duplex system, obstruction to flow due to a calculus, or a filling defect in the renal calyx, ureter or bladder.
- Aortography—the renal arteries may be defined by aortography. Stenosis of the renal artery or abnormal tumour circulation can be demonstrated. In selected cases renal artery arteriography can be combined with transluminal angioplasty for renal artery stenosis.
- CT scan—used to assess the local spread of renal tumours.
- Radionuclide scan—this can be used to demonstrate anatomical differences between the kidneys and provide dynamic imaging of the renal tract, particularly in the presence of urinary tract obstruction. Technetium-labelled diethylene triamine pentaacetic acid (DPTA) can provide information on renal perfusion, function, and the presence of obstruction. Technetium-labelled dimercaptosuccinic acid (DMSA) is taken up by the tubules and can be used to demonstrate the cortex and assess renal size and function.

Cystoscopy

The usual method for investigating the bladder is cystoscopy—rigid or flexible. It can usually be performed under local anaesthetic and sedation in the outpatient clinic. It allows direct visualization of the bladder and ureteric openings. Biopsies can be taken to assess suspicious lesions of the bladder mucosa.

Bladder neoplasms and the prostate can be resected via the cystoscope—transurethral resection of prostate (TURP) and transurethral resection of the tumour (TURT).

Ureteric calculi can be removed via ureteroscopes and dormia baskets passed via the cystoscope into the ureters.

A urethroscope is used to visualize the urethra.

Urodynamics

This is dynamic assessment of the storage and voiding function of the urinary tract.

Flow rate

Urine flow rate is measured to assess the rate and pattern of voiding.

Cystometry

This involves measurement of intravesical pressures during filling and voiding and is useful for differentiating between urge and stress incontinence.

Videocystometry

This involves filling the bladder with contrast medium during cystometry so that bladder activity can be observed on a fluoroscope during the filling and voiding phase.

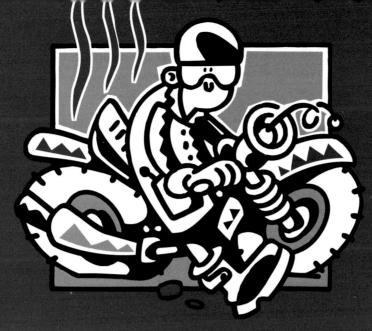

BACKGROUND INFORMATION
AND MANAGEMENT PLANS

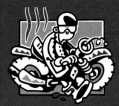

25. Oesophageal Disorders

The oesophagus extends from the pharynx to the gastric cardia and measures 25–30 cm in length. It has an upper sphincter, the cricopharyngeus, which is at the level of the sixth cervical vertebra and a lower sphincter derived from the inner circular muscle fibres of the oesophagus (40 cm from the incisors on endoscopy). The mucosal lining is squamous epithelium except for the lowest 2 cm, which is columnar epithelium.

The commonest symptoms of oesophageal disease are reflux and dysphagia.

GASTRO-OESOPHAGEAL REFLUX

Background

Normally, reflux of gastric contents is prevented by:
- The lower oesophageal sphincter.
- The angle of His.
- Crural fibres of the diaphragm.
- The prominent mucosal folds, which act as a plug.
- Positive intra-abdominal pressure acting on the lower oesophagus maintaining a high-pressure zone.

If these mechanisms fail or there is a hiatus hernia (i.e. a weakness in the diaphragm, which allows the stomach into the chest), either a sliding hiatus hernia or a paraoesophageal hernia then the gastric contents can reflux into the oesophagus, causing oesophagitis (Fig. 25.1).

Clinical presentation

The symptoms of reflux are:
- Retrosternal pain exacerbated by bending over or lying down.
- Regurgitation of acid into the mouth.
- Dysphagia if a stricture develops.

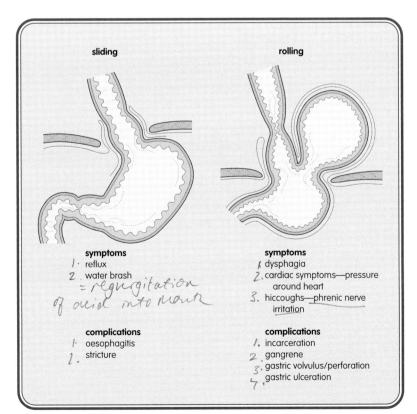

Fig. 25.1 Symptoms and complications of sliding and rolling hiatus hernias.

[handwritten top margin:] NO! When squamous oesophageal epi. repeatedly damaged by reflux → replaced by ectopic/metaplastic columnar epithelium.

Complications of reflux are:

1. • Oesophagitis—ulceration of the oesophageal mucosa ranging from mild to severe.
2. • Barrett's oesophagus—this is metaplastic change of the columnar epithelium to squamous epithelium *?? [handwritten]* and this may progress to dysplasia and malignant change.
3. • Barrett's ulcer—this can bleed or perforate.
4. • Iron deficiency anaemia—chronic blood loss from severe oesophagitis.
5. • Stricture—when oesophagitis heals it can develop into a fibrotic stricture, which causes dysphagia.
6. • Oesophageal cancer—this can develop in a long segment of Barrett's mucosa with dysplasia.

Management

Investigations include:

1. • Barium swallow—defines the anatomy of a hiatus hernia or stricture.
2. • Endoscopy and biopsy—direct visualization of damaged mucosa.
3. • pH monitoring and manometry—24-hour monitoring of pH and pressure.

Patients who have symptoms of reflux are given simple advice to avoid situations that exacerbate symptoms (i.e. sleep propped up, weight reduction, stop smoking, decrease intake of alcohol, caffeine, and spicy foods).

Medical treatment includes antacids and alginates, which provide a protective barrier on the gastric contents (Fig. 25.2).

• Gastric acid production can be decreased by histamine H_2-antagonists or proton pump inhibitors.

• Prokinetic drugs can increase the oesophageal motility and the tone of the sphincter.

Most people respond to medical treatment, but if there are any complications or the patient is young then surgical treatment is appropriate.

If the patient has a stricture it is dilated endoscopically by bougies and then a fundoplication can be performed laparoscopically or by open operation. The hiatus hernia is reduced and the fundus of the stomach is wrapped around the lower oesophagus and this increases the pressure to prevent reflux.

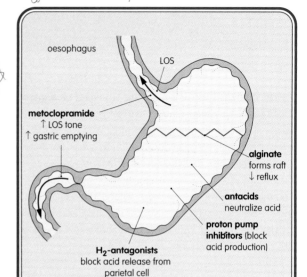

Fig. 25.2 Sites of action of drugs used to treat gastro-oesophageal reflux disease. (LOS, lower oesophageal sphincter.)

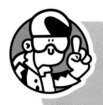

Patients who have a benign oesophageal stricture usually have a past history of gastro-oesophageal reflux.

BENIGN TUMOURS OF THE OESOPHAGUS

These are unusual, but the commonest is a leiomyoma, which causes dysphagia and can be removed from the submucosa to relieve symptoms.

OESOPHAGEAL CANCER

Background

Carcinoma is increasingly common in the Western World. It is more common in males, the male to female ratio being 3 to 1 and patients are usually over 50 years of age. There is a high incidence in China and South Africa.

Predisposing factors are:

- Barrett's oesophagus with dysplasia.
- Corrosive oesophagitis.
- Achalasia.
- Plummer–Vinson syndrome.
- Environmental factors, including smoking, alcohol, and dietary nitrosamines.

Carcinomas of the upper and middle thirds of the oesophagus are squamous cell carcinomas and those of the lower third are adenocarcinomas. The tumours spread locally and via the lymphatics and bloodstream.

Clinical presentation

The presenting symptoms include progressive dysphagia, iron deficiency anaemia, and weight loss (because many cases present late).

Management

Diagnosis and assessment of oesophageal cancer is made by:

- Barium swallow—enables assessment of the position and length of the stricture (Fig. 25.3).
- Endoscopy and biopsy—defines the histological type of tumour.
- Endoscopic ultrasound—provides accurate assessment of paraoesophageal disease and operability.
- Computed tomography (CT) scan of the chest and liver—to stage the tumour and assess any metastases.
- Bronchoscopy—may be performed if bronchial involvement is suspected.

Accurate assessment helps to plan treatment. If the tumour is operable and the patient is fit for a major thoracoabdominal operation then oesophageal resection with gastric or colonic interposition is the best symptomatic treatment. The role of chemotherapy and radiotherapy before operation is being assessed.

Many oesophageal carcinomas are inoperable so treatment is palliative. A squamous cell carcinoma of the upper and middle thirds will respond to radiotherapy. All tumours can be intubated with plastic or metal stents and lasers can be used to destroy the tumour to give some relief of dysphagia.

The prognosis is very poor. After resection 5-year survival is 15%, but overall 5-year survival is only 4%.

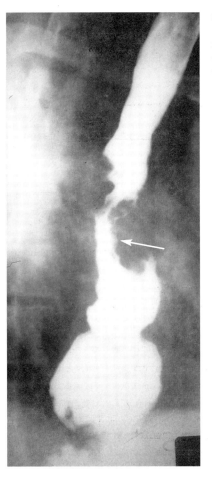

Fig. 25.3
Barium swallow showing oesophageal cancer (arrow).

Carcinoma of the lower one-third of the oesophagus is usually adenocarcinoma and the rest are squamous cell carcinomas.

ACHALASIA

Background

This condition is due to degeneration of the myenteric nerve plexus so that there is a failure of peristalsis and failure of relaxation of the lower oesophageal sphincter. It can present at any age, but usually between 30 and 60 years of age. It is more common in women, the male to female ratio being 2 to 3, and there is a risk of malignancy in the long term.

Clinical presentation

The usual symptoms are progressive dysphagia, weight loss, and aspiration pneumonia.

Management

The diagnosis is be made by:

- Chest radiography—may show a grossly dilated oesophagus with a fluid level and signs of aspiration pneumonia.
- Barium swallow—this will show a grossly dilated, tortuous oesophagus with a very narrow segment, 'rat tail', at the lower oesophageal sphincter (Fig. 25.4).
- Manometry—will demonstrate failure of relaxation of the sphincter.
- Endoscopy and biopsy—to detect malignant change.

Medical treatment is usually ineffective.

Pneumatic dilatation of the sphincter may give temporary relief, but operation (Heller's cardiomyotomy, which divides the lower oesophageal sphincter to the level of the mucosa) provides the best results.

Other motility disorders can produce dysphagia and retrosternal pain, which may simulate a myocardial infarction. Assessment includes a barium swallow and manometry, which will show the typical pattern of oesophageal contractions. These may be diffuse and uncoordinated or produce a corkscrew oesophagus (i.e. high-amplitude wave; Fig. 25.5). Therapy with long-acting nitrates and calcium channel blockers may be beneficial.

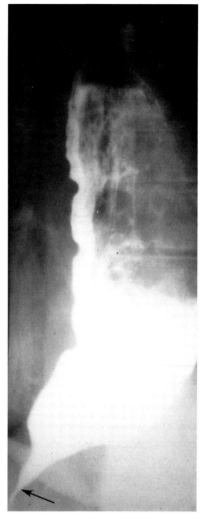

Fig. 25.4
Barium swallow showing achalasia. The oesophagus is dilated and there is a 'rat-tail' segment (arrow) at the lower oesophageal sphincter.

PHARYNGEAL POUCH

Background

Pharyngeal pouch (Fig. 25.6) is a condition of elderly people and it is more common in men than women. It is due to a mucosal protrusion between the parts of the inferior pharyngeal constrictor—the thyropharyngeus and the cricopharyngeus (i.e. Killian's dehiscence). It is thought to occur because of increased pressure developing when the upper oesophageal sphincter fails to relax.

Clinical presentation

The symptoms of a pharyngeal pouch are those of dysphagia, but with a characteristic 'double swallow' when the pouch empties. There may be a visible swelling in the neck. Regurgitation of the contents of the pouch may produce halitosis or recurrent aspiration pneumonia.

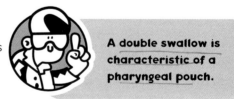

A double swallow is characteristic of a pharyngeal pouch.

Management

The diagnosis is made by the classic appearance of the pouch on a barium swallow. An endoscopy should not be performed because of the risk of perforation.

Treatment is operative excision of the pouch with a myotomy of the cricopharyngeus to prevent recurrence.

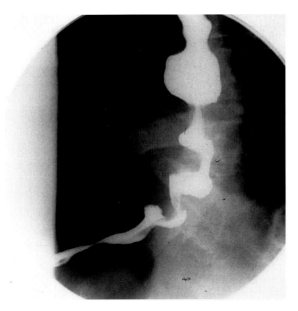

Fig. 25.5 Barium swallow showing typical contractions of a corkscrew oesophagus.

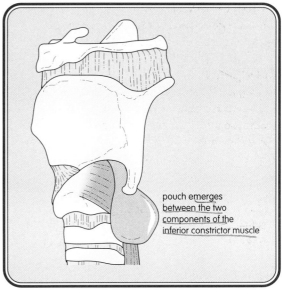

pouch emerges between the two components of the inferior constrictor muscle

Fig. 25.6 Anatomy of a pharyngeal pouch.

PLUMMER–VINSON SYNDROME

This occurs in middle-aged and elderly females. The syndrome consists of dysphagia and iron deficiency anaemia. The dysphagia is associated with hyperkeratinization of the oesophagus with formation of a web in the upper part. The condition is premalignant.

PERFORATION OF THE OESOPHAGUS

Background
This can occur:
- As a result of swallowing a foreign body.
- During oesophagoscopy and dilatation, especially if there is a malignant stricture.
- Spontaneously as a result of violent vomiting.

Clinical presentation
The symptoms are sudden onset of pain in the neck, chest, and abdomen. The patient may develop circulatory collapse, pyrexia, and surgical emphysema in the supraclavicular region of the neck.

Management
A chest radiograph may show mediastinal air, a pneumothorax, or fluid in the peritoneal cavity. A barium swallow confirms the site of rupture.

If the underlying problem is benign then surgical treatment is performed to resect or repair the damaged oesophagus. If the problem is due to malignancy and the patient is unfit for a major operation the patient is kept nil by mouth and intravenous fluids, antibiotics, and parenteral nutrition are prescribed. A chest drain is inserted.

The complications of perforation of the oesophagus are mediastinitis and empyema and there is a high mortality rate.

DYSPHAGIA

The differential diagnoses of dysphagia is detailed in Fig. 9.1, p. 37.

BASIC ANAT. + HISTOLOGY OF STOMACH.

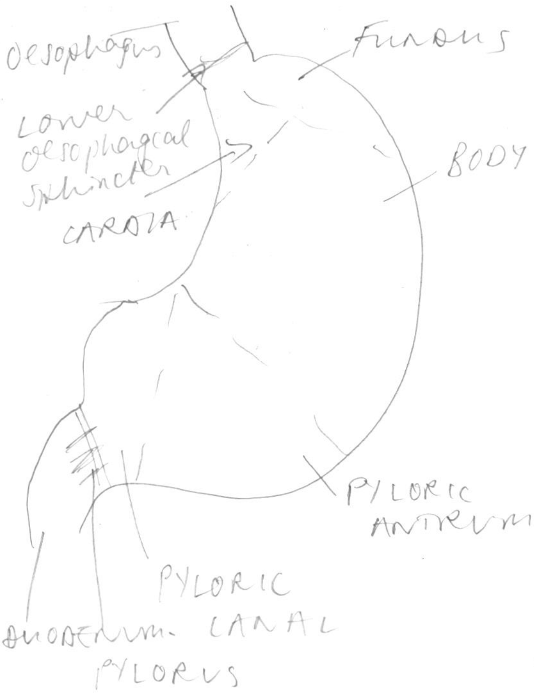

oesophagus

FUNDUS

Lower oesophageal sphincter

BODY

CARDIA

PYLORIC ANTRUM

DUODENUM

PYLORIC CANAL

PYLORUS

B.S STOMACH.

splenic art.

Coeliac axis

Short gastric

Hepatic art.

(R) gastric art.

(L) gastro-epiploic

gastro-duodenal art.

(R) gastro-epiploic

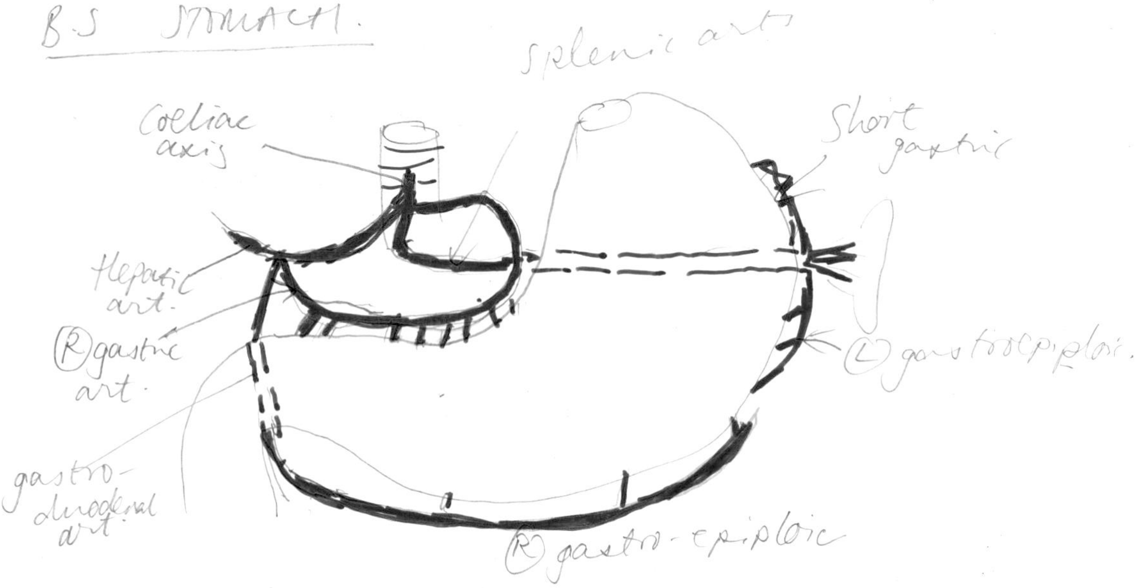

- Histology = simple columnar epithelium c̄ gastric glands wh contain exocrine glands

→ Upper 2/3 : ① Parietal cells → HCl
  ② Chief cells → Pepsinogen.

→ Antrum : G cells → gastrin → stimulates HCl release from parietal cells. (via histamine)

NB: Parietal cells secrete HCl in response to Ach, gastrin + histamine

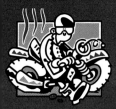

26. Gastric and Duodenal Disorders

The main function of the stomach is to act as a reservoir for ingested food. The upper part of the stomach is capable of adaptive relaxation to accommodate the food. The antrum acts as a mill and its contractions fulfil two functions:

- To churn the food into chyme.
- To deliver it in graduated amounts into the duodenum.

There is some digestion of the food by hydrochloric acid and pepsin.

Dyspepsia is a very common problem that is often treated by self-medication, but has several different causes, some of which are potentially serious.

PEPTIC ULCERATION

Background

There are several locations where ulceration can occur:

- Stomach.
- Duodenum.
- Oesophagus.
- Meckel's diverticulum in the terminal ileum.

Ulceration occurs where there is a breakdown in the mucosal defence mechanism, and may be associated with increased or inappropriate acid or pepsin secretion. Cytoprotective systems such as mucosal prostaglandin E_2 and mucosal bicarbonate secretion are both reduced in patients who have duodenal ulceration. These circumstances produce the right environment for the proteolytic enzyme pepsin to cause mucosal ulceration. There is also strong evidence for the involvement of the organism *Helicobacter pylori* in the aetiology of peptic ulceration. Other associations with peptic ulceration are:

- Smoking.
- Alcohol.
- Blood group O. — D u Bu ? G. u ↑ gp. A
- Non-steroidal anti-inflammatory drugs (NSAIDs).
- Corticosteroids.
- Stress.
- Hyperparathyroidism.
- Zollinger–Ellison syndrome (i.e. gastrinoma).

Classification of peptic ulceration

Peptic ulcers are classified into the following categories:

- Gastric ulcer type I—generally occurs on the lesser curve of the stomach.
- Gastric ulcer type II—occurs in the pyloric and prepyloric region and has the same features as duodenal ulcer.
- Duodenal ulcer—usually occurs in the first and second parts of the duodenum.

The features and presentation of gastric and duodenal ulcers are outlined in Fig. 26.1.

Clinical features of gastric and duodenal ulcers		
Feature	Duodenal ulcer	Gastric ulcer
Age	30–60 years	usually >50 years
Sex	m>f	m:f = 1:1
Epigastric pain	worse at night	worse after food
Associated features	relieved by food and antacids	vomiting and reflux, iron deficiency anaemia
Periodic pain	yes—attacks last 4–5 days followed by relief for a few weeks	no periodicity

Fig. 26.1 Clinical features of gastric and duodenal ulcers. (f, female; m, male.)

GD: 90% / Acid: ↑   80% / H. pylori Øve / Acid: ⟷

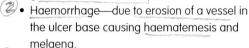
Complications of peptic ulceration

Complications associated with peptic ulceration are:

1. • Perforation—this will produce sudden onset of severe generalized abdominal pain.
2. • Haemorrhage—due to erosion of a vessel in the ulcer base causing haematemesis and melaena.
3. • Pyloric stenosis—when a duodenal or pyloric ulcer heals with scarring it can cause stenosis. The patient presents with progressive vomiting of undigested food, weight loss, dehydration, and hypokalaemic hypochloraemic alkalosis.
4. • Malignancy—only associated with gastric ulcers (1% of cases).
5. • Iron deficiency anaemia—may be presentation of peptic ulcer.

Management

g. u. only?

1. Diagnosis is made by gastroscopy. Biopsies are taken to assess for gastritis, malignancy, or *H. pylori* infection using the 'Clo test' (i.e. rapid urease test). Antibodies to *H. pylori* can be measured, but will reveal present and past infection.
2. Treatment of peptic ulcers is as follows:
   • Duodenal ulcers associated with *H. pylori* are treated with triple therapy (i.e. proton pump inhibitor, amoxycillin and metronidazole for 2 weeks). Treatment produces 80% eradication of infection and healing of ulcer.
   • Other medications to heal ulcers—either H_2-antagonists or proton pump inhibitors, which heal 90% of ulcers after 6–8 weeks of treatment.
   • Elective operation for duodenal ulceration—this is rarely required, but if it is a highly selective vagotomy is carried out. An operation may be required if a gastric ulcer fails to heal and this usually means a partial gastrectomy (i.e. excision of ulcer and antrum and restoration of gastroduodenal continuity).

Operations are required for the complications of peptic ulcers. These often occur in the elderly population and complications include:
• Perforation.
• Bleeding.
• Pyloric stenosis.

Diagnosis of perforation is made from a history of acute abdominal pain, signs of peritonitis, and free gas under the diaphragm on a chest radiograph. At laparotomy the perforation is oversewn with an omental patch. A gastric ulcer should be biopsied to exclude malignancy.

A diagnosis of bleeding is made at endoscopy and it may be possible to stop the bleeding by injecting the vessel with adrenaline or coagulating the vessel with a laser. If the bleeding recurs or continues the patient requires an emergency operation to under-run the vessel. If the ulcer is a duodenal ulcer this will be combined with a vagotomy and pyloroplasty (Fig. 26.2). A partial gastrectomy (see Fig. 26.2) may be needed to remove a gastric ulcer.

The initial management of pyloric stenosis is to correct the fluid and electrolyte imbalance. A subsequent vagotomy and gastroenterostomy is required to bypass the pyloric obstruction (see Fig. 26.2).

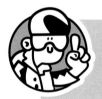

Patients who have a gastric ulcer need a repeat endoscopy 6–8 weeks later to make sure that the ulcer has healed.

Many patients have had a gastric operation in the past and still experience the side effects of the operation such as:

1. • Steatorrhoea and diarrhoea. *(intestinal hurry)*
2. • Dumping—the symptoms of fainting, vertigo, and sweating, which may be due to the osmotic effect of rapid transit of food from the stomach into the small intestine after pyloroplasty or gastric surgery. Fluid is absorbed into the jejunum causing temporary hypovolaemia.
3. • Bile reflux and vomiting.
4. • Small stomach syndrome.
5. • Anaemia—may be due to iron deficiency because hydrochloric acid is required for iron absorption or due to vitamin B_{12} deficiency because intrinsic factor is required. Both hydrochloric acid and intrinsic factor are absent after partial gastrectomy.
6. • Stomal ulceration.
7. • Malignancy in the gastric remnant.
8. *Blind loop syndrome*
9. *Osteomalacia – malab. of Vit. D + Ca²⁺.*

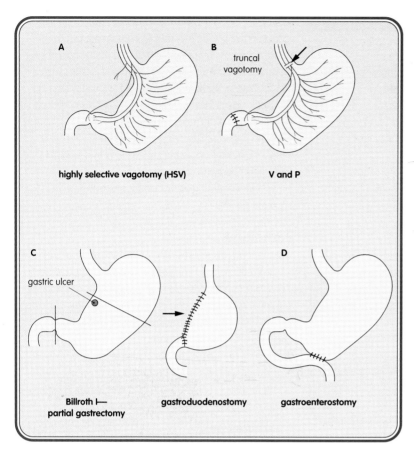

Fig. 26.2 Gastric operations. **(A)** In highly selective vagotomy the branches of the vagus nerve innervating the parietal cells are divided to decrease gastric acid secretion. **(B)** In vagotomy and pyloroplasty (V and P) the main vagal trunks are divided (arrow) to decrease gastric acid secretion. Pyloroplasty is required to overcome the impaired gastric contraction that results. **(C)** Partial gastrectomy for gastric ulcer. **(D)** Gastroenterostomy.

EROSIVE GASTRITIS

Background
Erosive gastritis is a common problem with several causes, including NSAIDs and critical illness.

Clinical presentation
In erosive gastritis there is often diffuse oedema and erythema of the gastric mucosa with focal mucosal haemorrhage, erosions, and ulceration. The condition may present with haematemesis.

CHRONIC ATROPHIC GASTRITIS

Chronic atrophic gastritis may be categorized into two types:
• Type A is associated with achlorrhydria, impaired absorption of vitamin B_{12}, the presence of parietal cell antibodies in serum, and the development of pernicious anaemia.

• Type B is caused by chronic mucosal damage (e.g. by dietary salts, viral infections, bile reflux, *H. pylori* infection). The gastritis may undergo metaplasia to intestinal-type epithelium and subsequently develop dysplasia and may progress to carcinoma.

ZOLLINGER–ELLISON SYNDROME

Background
This is intractable gastroduodenal ulceration caused by
• Gastrin secretion.
• An amine precursor uptake and decarboxylation (APUD) tumour, which is commonly found in the pancreas and can be benign or malignant.

Management
Diagnosis is made by measuring serum gastrin levels. Treatment is by use of a proton pump inhibitor or resection if it is a solitary tumour.

127

GASTRIC CANCER

Background

Gastric tumours can be benign or malignant, but cancer is more common. Benign tumours include:

- Adenomas—epithelial polyps.
- Leiomyoma.
- Fibroma.
- Neurofibroma.
- Haemangioma.

Malignant tumours include:

- Adenocarcinoma (most common).
- Leiomyosarcoma and lymphoma.

Gastric cancer is the third commonest gastrointestinal cancer in the UK. Its incidence is declining, but there seems to be an increasing incidence of cardia tumours since the introduction of H_2-antagonists. It tends to present late in the UK and has a poor prognosis. The peak age is 70–80 years and it is more common in males than in females.

In other parts of the world (e.g. Japan), there is a high incidence of gastric cancer and there are screening programmes to detect it early. Risk factors for development of gastric cancer are outlined in Fig. 26.3.

Pathology

The macroscopic morphology of gastric cancer is shown in Fig. 26.4. Early gastric cancer comprises a nodule or ulceration confined to the mucosa and submucosa, but in the UK most of the gastric cancers have invaded the muscularis propria at the time of presentation to produce any of the following:

- Malignant ulcer with raised everted edges.
- Polypoid tumour (proliferating mucosa protruding into the lumen).
- Colloid tumour (a gelatinous growth).
- Linitis plastica (submucous infiltration by cancer cells, resulting in a marked fibrotic reaction and the

---

Risk factors for development of gastric cancer
atrophic gastritis
blood group A
pernicious anaemia
adenomatous polyps
diet—spicy, salty foods, excess nitrates
smoking
alcohol
Helicobacter pylori infection

Fig. 26.3 Risk factors for the development of gastric cancer.

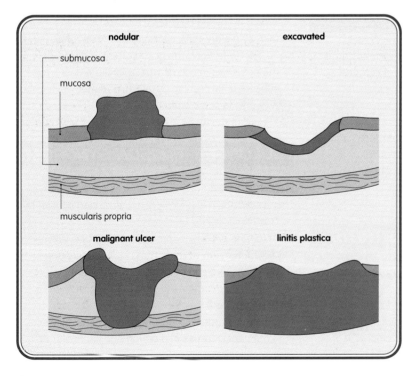

Fig. 26.4 Growth patterns of gastric cancer.

nodular

excavated

submucosa

mucosa

muscularis propria

malignant ulcer

linitis plastica

stomach is contracted and thickened with little mucosal ulceration).

Most gastric cancers are adenocarcinomas and they are defined as intestinal or diffuse:

- Intestinal cancers arise on a background of atrophic gastritis and are well-circumscribed adenocarcinomas.
- Diffuse cancer arises from a 'normal' stomach and is a poorly localized lesion that infiltrates rapidly into the submucosa. It spreads locally to invade adjacent structures such as the liver, pancreas, and transverse colon.

Lymphatic spread is to the nodes along the lesser and greater curvatures of the stomach, to the coeliac axis, hepatic nodes, and then to the supraclavicular nodes via the thoracic duct.

Bloodstream spread is via the portal system to the liver and subsequently to the lungs.

Transcoelomic spread produces peritoneal seedlings and Krukenberg's tumours (i.e. secondary tumours in the ovaries).

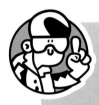

If a patient has an enlarged left supraclavicular node of Virchow (i.e. Troisier's sign) look for intra-abdominal pathology.

Clinical presentation

A diagnosis of gastric cancer should be suspected if there is:

- Recent onset of dyspepsia.
- Dysphagia—due to obstruction of the gastro-oesophageal junction.
- Vomiting—may be due to pyloric outlet obstruction.
- Anorexia and weight loss.
- Iron deficiency anaemia.
- Abdominal swelling due to ascites, mass, or hepatomegaly.
- Metastatic disease (e.g. jaundice).

- Virchow's node = Troisier's sign in ① supraclavicular fossa.

The diagnosis is confirmed by gastroscopy and biopsy. Additional assessment and staging can be made by:

- Blood tests (e.g. full blood count, liver function tests).
- Chest radiography.
- Hepatic ultrasound—to look for metastases.
- Computed tomography (CT) scan of abdomen—to assess nodal disease and involvement of adjacent structures.
- Laparoscopy—to assess operability and look for peritoneal seedlings and serosal disease, which is not seen on a CT scan.

Management

If the tumour is resectable and confined to the stomach gastric resection and radical resection of the drainage lymph nodes gives the best long-term results. Antral tumours are treated by subtotal gastrectomy, but carcinoma of the upper stomach is treated by a total gastrectomy with Roux-en-Y loop reconstruction using small intestine anastomosed to the oesophagus.

If the tumour is unresectable, palliative surgery may be a gastroenterostomy for pyloric outlet obstruction or insertion of a stent for carcinoma of the gastro-oesophageal junction or cardia. The role of chemotherapy is still unproven.

The prognosis is very poor. After 'curative' resection the 5-year survival rates are only 20% except for early gastric cancer; overall 5-year survival is about 5%.

GASTRIC LYMPHOMA

The stomach is the commonest site of primary extranodal lymphoma, but gastric lymphoma is still rare. It arises from the mucosa associated lymphoid tissue (MALT) and *H. pylori* has also been implicated.

Clinical presentation

The symptoms of gastric lymphoma are those of gastric cancer.

Management

Treatment is by resection if possible, followed by radiotherapy. Non-resectable tumours can be treated by combination chemotherapy and radiotherapy. The prognosis is better than for adenocarcinoma.

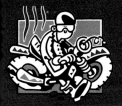

27. Disorders of Small Intestine

The main function of the small intestine is digestion and absorption of nutrients (fats, carbohydrates, and proteins). This occurs in the jejunum and the upper ileum. Bile salts and vitamin B_{12} are absorbed from the terminal ileum.

OBSTRUCTION OF THE SMALL INTESTINE

Background
A common cause for acute surgical admission is small bowel obstruction. The speed of the onset can be acute, chronic, or acute on chronic.

Clinical presentation
The presenting symptoms are colicky abdominal pain, vomiting, absolute constipation, and abdominal distension. The cause may be:

- In the lumen—tumour (e.g. leiomyoma), food bolus, gall stone.
- In the wall—Crohn's disease, radiation stricture.
- Outside the lumen—adhesions, volvulus, hernia, intussusception.

The most common causes are adhesions and irreducible hernias.

Management
The diagnosis is made from the history and clinical examination, which includes making a note of:

- Hydration.
- Pulse.
- Blood pressure.
- Temperature.
- Mucous membranes.
- Abdominal scars.
- Hernial orifices.
- Distension.
- Presence of high-pitched bowel sounds.

Any signs of tenderness or peritonism imply that the bowel may be getting ischaemic.

Investigations should include:
- Full blood count—may demonstrate an elevated white cell count.
- Renal function.
- Abdominal radiograph—may show small bowel dilatation.

Treatment is by resuscitation with intravenous fluids, monitoring the pulse, blood pressure, and urine output. A nasogastric tube is passed to prevent vomiting and decompress the bowel.

Urgent surgical intervention is required if the patient has a tender incarcerated hernia or any signs of peritonism.

If the patient has had a previous operation adhesions are the likely cause and the patient is initially treated conservatively for 24 hours if he or she has no signs of peritonism. If the condition fails to resolve a laparotomy is required.

CROHN'S DISEASE

Background
Crohn's disease is a chronic inflammatory bowel disease. It can affect any part of the alimentary tract from the mouth to the anus, but particularly the small intestine (Fig. 27.1). Its aetiology is obscure. Crohn's disease occurs more commonly in females, the male to female ratio being 1 to 1.6, and is usually diagnosed in young adults.

Pathology
Macroscopically, the bowel looks red, oedematous, and thickened in Crohn's disease. The mesentery is thickened and the fat encroaches on the bowel wall. The lesions are intermittent (i.e. skip lesions). In the mucosa there are deep ulcers—'rose thorn ulcer' and there is cobblestone mucosa. Microscopically there is transmural inflammation, which may include the presence of non-caseating granulomas.

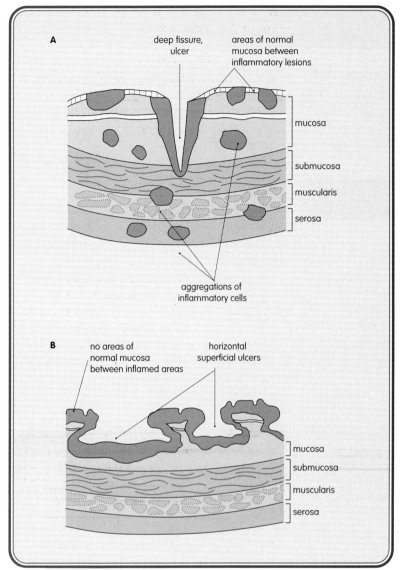

Fig. 27.1 (A) Pathological features of Crohn's disease, showing mucosal ulceration. Compare this with the features of ulcerative colitis (which affects the colon and rectum, see p. 138) and shown in **(B)** in which there is transmural inflammation with deep ulceration.

A

deep fissure, ulcer

areas of normal mucosa between inflammatory lesions

mucosa

submucosa

muscularis

serosa

aggregations of inflammatory cells

B

no areas of normal mucosa between inflamed areas

horizontal superficial ulcers

mucosa

submucosa

muscularis

serosa

Clinical presentation

The patient may present with:

- Abdominal pain.
- Change of bowel habit and nausea.
- Weight loss.
- Anaemia.
- Malnutrition.

Crohn's disease may cause perianal problems such as perianal sepsis, fistulae, fissures, or skin tags.

The initial presentation of Crohn's disease often results from involvement of the terminal ileum and after resection many people have no further problems, but in some people Crohn's disease is a chronic recurring disease with long-term morbidity.

Extraintestinal manifestations of Crohn's disease include:

- Uveitis.
- Episcleritis of the eye.
- Arthritis.
- Aphthous ulcers.
- Erythema nodosum.

Complications include strictures causing acute or chronic intestinal obstruction. Abscesses may be perianal or intraperitoneal (between the loops of intestine), and fistulae may be enteroenteric, enterocutaneous, or vesicocolic.

Management
Diagnosis of Crohn's disease is made by demonstrating:
• Iron deficiency anaemia.
• Elevated erythrocyte sedimentation rate and C-reactive protein.

A small bowel enema will demonstrate Kantor's string sign of a stricture, 'rose- thorn' ulcers, and fissures.
An ultrasound may be helpful in assessing intraperitoneal abdominal masses related to Crohn's disease.
Treatment is initially with:
• Corticosteroids.
• Sulphasalazine.
• Immunosuppressive agents such as azathioprine.

Surgical operations are reserved for complications and limited resections are performed because there is a high risk of further problems. If there is a fibrotic stricture a stricturoplasty is performed.
In the long term Crohn's disease is chronic so there is a risk of developing short bowel syndrome.

SHORT GUT SYNDROME

This follows massive resection of the small intestine. Common causes are:
• Mesenteric infarction.
• Crohn's disease.
• Radiation enteritis.

The critical length of small intestine needed to maintain nutrition is 1–2 m. After resection the remaining intestine adapts by dilatation of the small intestine and villous enlargement to improve absorption. If there is less than 1 m and oral nutrition is inadequate total parenteral nutrition is necessary.

INTESTINAL ISCHAEMIA

Background
Acute ischaemia of the small intestine can be caused by a fall in cardiac output or vascular occlusion due to embolus or thrombosis of the superior mesenteric artery or vein. These may be associated with atherosclerosis or atrial fibrillation.

Clinical presentation
There is a history of sudden onset of severe abdominal pain. On examination the patient is unwell with increased pulse rate, decreased blood pressure, and generalized abdominal tenderness.

Management
The diagnosis is based upon:
• Clinical suspicion.
• Elevated white cell count.
• Acidosis.

Treatment is by resuscitation and a laparotomy. If the whole of the small intestine is infarcted it is not appropriate to resect because the patient is unlikely to survive. If part of the bowel is affected then a resection is performed, but it is not anastomosed because of the risk of further ischaemia. The ends of the intestine are brought to the surface as stomas. It is often not possible to perform an embolectomy.

Suspect ischaemic bowel if the patient's symptoms are more marked than the physical signs.

CHRONIC ISCHAEMIA

Background
Chronic ischaemia is due to atherosclerosis of the superior mesenteric artery.

Clinical presentation
The symptoms of chronic ischaemia are colicky abdominal pain after eating. The patient is afraid to eat so there is malnutrition and weight loss.

Management
A diagnosis of chronic ischaemia is made by arteriograms. It may be possible to insert a stent or perform a bypass operation.

RADIATION ENTEROPATHY

Background

Radiotherapy may damage the small and large intestine. It causes proliferative endarteritis and vasculitis, resulting in ischaemia and transmural fibrosis. Patients who have diabetes mellitus, hypertension, and cardiovascular disease are more prone to the complications of radiotherapy.

Clinical presentation

The symptoms are usually:
- Chronic abdominal pain.
- Diarrhoea.
- Rectal bleeding.

Complications include haemorrhage, perforation, and obstruction.

MECKEL'S DIVERTICULUM

Background

Meckel's diverticulum is the remnant of the vitellointestinal duct of the embryo and lies on the antimesenteric border of the ileum. It occurs in 2% of people, 60 cm (2 ft) from the ileocaecal valve and is about 5 cm (2 in) in length. It may contain heterotopic tissue (gastric, duodenal, or pancreatic).

Meckel's diverticulum is a true diverticulum and consists of all intestinal layers.

Clinical presentation

Most Meckel's diverticula are asymptomatic, but clinical presentations can result from:
- Acute inflammation—which may simulate acute appendicitis.
- Presence of gastric mucosa—this carries a risk of ulceration causing bleeding and or perforation. Meckel's diverticulum is a common cause of bleeding in children. The problem can be diagnosed by a technetium-labelled red cell scan if it is bleeding.
- Intussusception—this will cause intermittent right-sided abdominal pain with an intermittent mass.
- Obstruction to the small intestine by a vitellointestinal band extending from the Meckel's diverticulum to the umbilicus.

Management

Management of Meckel's diverticulum is by surgical excision if a complication occurs.

INTUSSUSCEPTION

Background

Intussusception in infants and young children may be due to a viral infection causing hyperplasia of the lymphoid tissue, which then acts as the apex of the intussusception. In older children or adults a polyp, carcinoma, or Meckel's diverticulum may be the apex. The inner layer of the intussusception has its blood supply cut off by pressure and stretching of the mesentery, so there is a risk of gangrene. A radiograph of intussuception is shown in Fig. 27.2.

Clinical presentation

In infants the history of intussusception comprises paroxysms of colic and the child screams. There is associated pallor, vomiting, and passage of redcurrant stool. A mass may be palpable in the right iliac fossa. Adults have a history suggestive of intestinal obstruction.

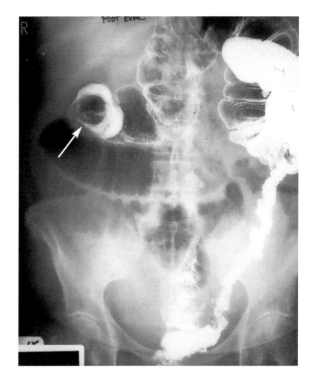

Fig. 27.2 Intussusception. Barium enema showing an ileocolic intussusception (arrow).

Management

If detected early in infants then the hydrostatic pressure of a barium enema may reduce an intussusception, but if there are signs of peritonism or a long history then operative intervention is required. If the bowel is gangrenous it is resected.

TUMOURS OF THE SMALL INTESTINE

Background

Tumours of the small intestine are rare and the following conditions are benign:

- Adenomas in familial polyposis.
- Gardner's syndrome (familial polyposis and cysts).
- Peutz–Jeghers syndrome (polyps and skin pigmentation).
- Lipomas.
- Leiomyomas.

The malignant tumours include adenocarcinoma, carcinoid tumours, leiomyosarcomas, lymphomas, or secondary deposits (e.g. melanoma). Small intestinal tumours tend to present late with intestinal obstruction.

CARCINOID TUMOURS

Background

These are neuroendocrine amine precursor uptake and decarboxylation system (APUD) tumours that arise from Kulchitsky's cells. They can arise anywhere in the intestinal tract and lungs, but commonly in the appendix. The foregut and midgut tumours secrete serotonin (also known as 5-hydroxytryptamine).

Clinical presentation

The primary tumour may produce symptoms of:

- Intestinal obstruction.
- Diarrhoea.
- Haemorrhage.

When the tumours metastasize to the liver the patient develops carcinoid syndrome, which is characterized by:

- Cutaneous flushing.
- Skin rashes.
- Intestinal colic.
- Diarrhoea.
- Bronchospasm.
- Cardiac lesions (tricuspid incompetence).
- Pulmonary stenosis.

Management

The diagnosis is made by urinary estimation of 5-hydroxyindoleacetic acid (5-HIAA), which is a derivative of serotonin.

Treatment is by:

- Resection, if possible.
- Embolization of hepatic metastases.
- Control of symptoms by long-acting somatostatin.

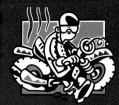

28. Colonic Disorders

ACUTE APPENDICITIS

Background

Acute appendicitis is a very common reason for acute surgical admission. It can occur at any age, but is most common in young children and young adults.

Acute appendicitis is thought to be due to luminal obstruction of the appendix with superimposed infection. Obstruction may be by a faecolith or swollen lymphoid follicles after a viral infection. Ulceration of the mucosa occurs and infection with mixed anaerobes and coliforms supervenes. The bacteria proliferate and invade the appendix wall, which is damaged by pressure necrosis.

The blood supply to the appendix is via an end-artery and when it is thrombosed gangrene develops. An acutely inflamed appendix may:

- Resolve spontaneously, especially if it is not obstructed, but may recur.
- Become gangrenous and perforate.
- Become surrounded by omentum and loops of bowel to wall off the infection and an appendix mass develops.

Clinical presentation

The illness starts as a mild periumbilical colicky pain followed by anorexia, nausea, and vomiting. A few hours later the pain becomes localized to the right iliac fossa. It is a constant pain exacerbated by movement. Diarrhoea may occur if the appendix is retroileal and dysuria may occur if it is pelvic.

On examination the patient may be flushed and have a pyrexia, tachycardia, and foetor.

On abdominal examination there is peritonism in the right iliac fossa. If the appendix is perforated the signs of peritonitis are more widespread.

Rectal examination demonstrates right-sided tenderness if the appendix is pelvic. If the symptoms have been present for 4 or 5 days an appendix mass may be present.

Fig. 28.1 shows the clinical progression of acute appendicitis.

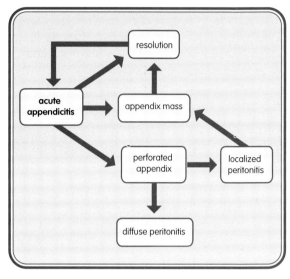

Fig. 28.1 Clinical progression of acute appendicitis.

Management

Diagnosis of acute appendicitis is made from the history and examination. There is usually a leucocytosis, but this is not specific. An ultrasound examination will demonstrate an appendix mass and ovarian pathology, but does not prove acute appendicitis.

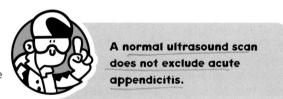

A normal ultrasound scan does not exclude acute appendicitis.

Treatment of acute appendicitis is emergency appendicectomy.

An appendix mass it is treated with intravenous antibiotics and fluids. The patient is monitored closely in case peritonitis develops, but if it resolves an elective appendicectomy is performed to prevent recurrence.

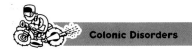

APPENDIX TUMOURS

Background

The appendix is occasionally the site of a tumour such as adenocarcinoma, mucinous neoplasm, and lymphoma. The appendix is, however, the commonest site for a carcinoid tumour. They are usually found incidentally at the tip of the organ and rarely metastasize, and the prognosis is good.

INFLAMMATORY BOWEL DISEASES

These are ulcerative colitis and Crohn's disease (see Chapter 27, Fig. 27.1). When affecting the colon these conditions produce similar symptoms, but it is important to distinguish between the two because of their different management and prognosis.

ULCERATIVE COLITIS

Background

Ulcerative colitis affects the colon, commencing from the rectum and proceeding continuously proximally. Its aetiology is obscure, but it may be associated with HLA-B27 and it usually presents in people who are aged 20–40 years. It is more common in females.

Macroscopically the mucosa is inflamed, oedematous, ulcerated, bleeding and producing mucous. Pseudopolyps may be seen (i.e. islands of normal mucosa between denuded areas).

Microscopically there is an inflammatory infiltrate in the mucosa and submucosa. The crypts of Lieberkühn are inflamed and crypt abscesses develop, coalesce, and cause ulceration.

Clinical presentation

Ulcerative colitis may have a mild and chronic course if it is confined to the distal colon and rectum. The symptoms are:
- Diarrhoea with passage of blood and mucus.
- Abdominal pain.
- Systemic symptoms of anorexia, low-grade pyrexia, and weight loss.

- Non-gastrointestinal symptoms include iritis, arthritis, sacroileitis, ankylosing spondylitis, pyoderma and erythema nodosum, renal calculi, pyelonephritis, hepatic disease, and cholangitis.

Ulcerative colitis may have an acute or acute on chronic presentation as toxic megacolon. The clinical features are:
- Profuse diarrhoea and rectal bleeding.
- Rapid development of hypovolaemia, tachycardia, pyrexia, and hypotension.
- Distended and tender abdomen with absent bowel sounds.

Management

A diagnosis of ulcerative colitis is made by:
- Sigmoidoscopy—showing the characteristic appearance of ulcerated, bleeding mucosa, and biopsies are taken to confirm the diagnosis and differentiate from Crohn's disease.
- Barium enema—to assess the extent of the disease—the characteristic changes are loss of the haustrations, and rigidity and shortening of the colon leading to a 'lead pipe' appearance.
- Abdominal radiography in the acute situation—may show signs of perforation or gross dilatation of toxic megacolon.

The complications of ulcerative colitis are toxic megacolon and carcinoma. Those patients who have had extensive colitis for more than 10 years are at increased risk of developing carcinoma so should have regular colonoscopy and biopsy to assess for dysplasia.

Treatment may consist of:
- Prednisolone enemas or sulphasalazine orally and by enemas—for mild short-segment disease.
- Systemic corticosteroids—for more severe episodes.
- Immunosuppressants such as azathioprine.
- Surgical operation—if medical treatment fails or complications develop, ulcerative colitis can be eradicated by performing a panproctocolectomy (removing the anus, rectum, and colon) and forming a permanent ileostomy. Alternatively the terminal ileum can be used to create an ileal pouch, which is anastomosed to the anus. Stool frequency is high and continence may be a problem so the patients need to be well motivated.

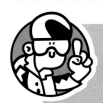

A common exam question is 'Discuss the differences between Crohn's disease and ulcerative colitis'.

CROHN'S DISEASE OF THE COLON

Background
The pathology of Crohn's disease of the colon is the same as for the small intestine (see Fig. 27.1).

Clinical presentation
Crohn's disease of the colon may present with:
- Abdominal pain.
- Diarrhoea.
- Rectal bleeding.
- Mucus discharge.
- Perianal problems.

Management
Treatment of Crohn's disease of the colon is similar to that of ulcerative colitis except that a panproctocolectomy does not cure the problem and a pouch is not created because of the risk of further disease in the ileum of the pouch (see Chapter 27).

DIVERTICULOSIS

Background
This is common in developed countries, but most people are asymptomatic. The incidence rises with increasing age and it is unusual in people under 40 years of age.

Diverticula develop when the diet is poor in fibre. As a result the segmental contractions of the colon are more vigorous and prolonged, increasing the intraluminal pressure, which leads to herniation of the mucosa between the taenia coli, giving rise to two rows of diverticula adjacent to the appendices epiploicae. They are pseudodiverticula because they consist only of mucosa and submucosa.

Diverticula are predominantly found in the sigmoid colon, but they can occur anywhere in the colon, including the caecum where caecal diverticulitis may mimic appendicitis.

Clinical presentation
Clinical presentations of diverticulosis are:
- Diverticulosis itself—episodes of left iliac fossa pain associated with alternating diarrhoea and constipation.
- *Acute diverticulitis—the patient is systemically unwell with pyrexia, tenderness, and peritonism in the left iliac fossa.
- Perforation—diverticulitis may proceed to perforation. If the infection is contained locally it causes a paracolic abscess, but if not it may cause generalized peritonitis.
- Fistula formation—in acute inflammation the colon may become adherent to the bladder, vagina, or small intestine. A vesicocolic fistula causes cystitis and pneumaturia. A colovaginal fistula causes a faeculent vaginal discharge.
- Obstruction—acute inflammation may narrow the lumen of the colon and repeated episodes cause thickening of the bowel wall and a fibrous stricture may develop, which causes episodes of subacute obstruction.
- Haemorrhage—erosion of a vessel at the mouth of a diverticulum may cause significant rectal bleeding.

Management
Diverticulosis is usually diagnosed by a barium enema, but if a complication occurs (Fig. 28.2) it may be found at laparotomy. The management of different stages is as follows:
- Diverticulosis—advice about a high fibre diet.
- Acute diverticulitis—most cases settle with intravenous fluids and intravenous antibiotics.
- Peritonitis—resuscitation, intravenous antibiotics, and fluids before a laparotomy, resection of the diseased segment of colon, and formation of a colostomy.
- Paracolic abscess—an ultrasound or CT scan may demonstrate a collection, which may be drained percutaneously or may require a laparotomy.
- Diverticular stricture—if recurrent episodes of subacute obstruction occur it may be necessary to resect the involved colon with a primary anastomosis.

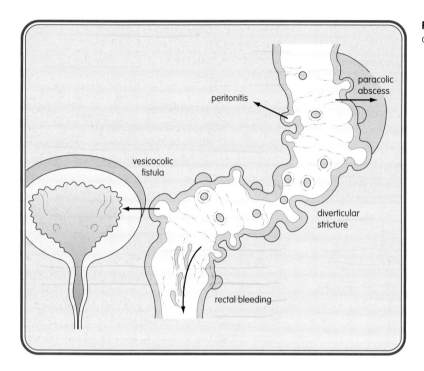

Fig. 28.2 Complications of diverticulosis.

- Fistula—elective resection of diseased colon, closure of fistula, and primary anastomosis.
- Diverticular haemorrhage—the initial management is resuscitation. Most cases settle spontaneously, but if not an arteriogram is performed to locate the site of bleeding so that the appropriate segment of colon is resected.

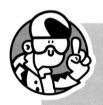

Complications of diverticulosis are acute diverticulitis, perforation, fistula formation, obstruction, and haemorrhage.

VOLVULUS

This is a twisting of a loop of bowel around its mesentery. It commonly occurs in the sigmoid colon, but can occur in the caecum or small intestine. It causes obstruction of the bowel and the blood supply is obstructed causing ischaemia and infarction.

Sigmoid volvulus
Background
This usually affects elderly patients who may be institutionalized and have a history of chronic constipation.

Clinical presentation
The symptoms are:
- Colicky abdominal pain.
- Absolute constipation.
- Gross abdominal distension.

Management
An abdominal radiograph shows the characteristic appearance of a grossly dilated sigmoid colon (Fig. 28.3). In some cases it can be decompressed using a rigid sigmoidoscope, but if it is a recurrent problem it should be resected electively. If it cannot be decompressed or there are signs of peritonism a laparotomy and resection are performed.

Caecal volvulus
Background
Caecal volvulus occurs if there is a congenital abnormality so that the caecum has a long mesentery and the caecum is mobile.

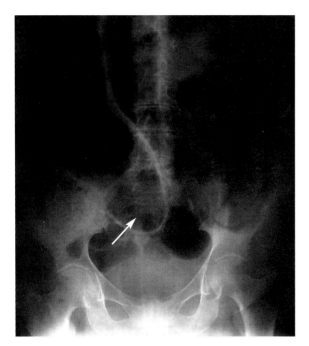

Fig. 28.3 Abdominal radiograph of sigmoid volvulus showing a grossly distended sigmoid loop (arrow).

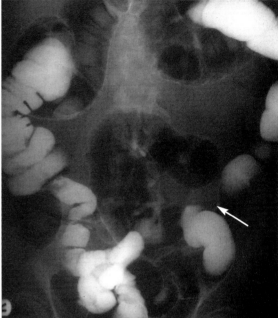

Fig. 28.4 Barium enema showing a polyp in the distal sigmoid colon.

Clinical presentation

The torsion causes an acute closed loop obstruction so the patient has symptoms of bowel obstruction or peritonitis if the caecum infarcts.

Management

Urgent laparotomy and colonic resection is required.

PSEUDO-OBSTRUCTION

Background

Pseudo-obstruction affects the elderly and infirm and is often associated with prolonged medical illnesses, including:

- Uraemia.
- Chronic lung disease.
- Immobility, especially after orthopaedic surgery.

Management

A diagnosis of pseudo-obstruction is made by the characteristic abdominal radiograph appearances of dilated small and large bowel loops. If a limited barium enema is performed it will flow freely into a dilated colon and there will be no signs of an obstructing lesion.

Treatment is conservative and most cases resolve. Electrolyte abnormalities such as hypokalaemia should be corrected because they can exacerbate the problem. Decompression by a colonoscopy is occasionally effective.

COLONIC POLYPS

Background

A polyp projects into the lumen of the bowel and is composed of epithelial and connective tissue elements. They occur anywhere in the bowel, but particularly in the colon and rectum (Fig. 28.4). Polyps can be:

- Neoplastic (i.e. adenomatous or villous papillomas).
- Inflammatory.
- Hamartomatous.

There are several syndromes associated with polyps:

- Familial polyposis coli—an autosomal dominant condition in which hundreds of adenomas develop through the colon and rectum during the second decade of life. They may be asymptomatic or cause rectal bleeding and diarrhoea, but there is a 100% risk of malignancy in 15 years.

Modified Dukes' classification of colorectal tumours		
Stage	Definition	5-year survival (%)
A	confined to the mucosa	90
B1	involves part of muscle wall	70
B2	reaches the serosa	60
C1	involves wall, but not completely; local lymph nodes involved	30
C2	involves serosa and lymph nodes	30

Fig. 28.5 Modified Dukes' classification of colorectal tumours.

- Gardner's syndrome—multiple colonic adenomas associated with sebaceous and dermoid cysts, osteomas, and desmoid tumours of the abdominal wall. There is a high risk of malignant change.

VILLOUS ADENOMA

Background
Villous adenoma is a sessile lesion that secretes large amounts of mucus and may produce diarrhoea and cause hypokalaemia. It carries a risk of developing dysplasia and malignant change.

Villous adenoma can be a cause of hypokalaemia.

COLONIC CARCINOMA

Background
Colonic carcinoma occurs in both sexes and is very common in the UK. Variation in incidence between different countries probably reflects dietary differences, particularly between developed and developing countries. A low fibre diet causes a long transit time and therefore greater exposure to any carcinogens. Other risk factors include:
- Familial polyposis coli.
- Ulcerative colitis.

- Adenomatous polyps.
- Gardner's syndrome.

Pathologically colonic carcinomas are adenocarcinomas, which can be:
- Polypoid.
- Ulcerative.
- Annular.
- Diffuse.
- Infiltrating.

The tumour invades the bowel wall and then spreads to the adjacent lymph nodes and the bloodstream. Approximately 3% of tumours are synchronous (i.e. two tumours at the same time), and 3% are metachronous. Fig. 28.5 shows the modifed Dukes' classification of colorectal tumours.

Clinical presentation
The symptoms of colorectal carcinoma depend upon its position in the colon and rectum.

Management
A diagnosis of colorectal carcinoma is made by:
- Clinical examination.
- Rigid sigmoidoscopy.
- Barium enema.
  + colonoscopy → ? any synchronous tumours.

A colonic carcinoma has a characteristic appearance of an 'apple core' on barium enema (Fig. 28.6). Colonoscopy can also be used and biopsies can be taken and any other polyps excised.

Blood tests such as a full blood count may show anaemia. Liver function tests and carcinoembryonic

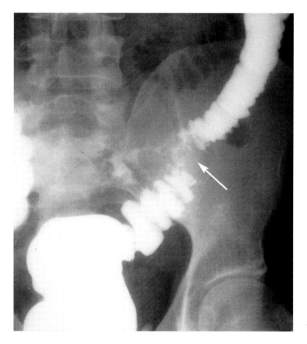

Fig. 28.6 Barium enema showing the 'apple-core' appearance (arrow) that is typical of carcinoma of the sigmoid colon.

antigen are measured to assess and monitor any metastatic disease. A computed tomography (CT) scan of the pelvis may be used to assess operability of a rectal cancer.

Fig. 28.7 shows the different presentations of colonic cancer.

Treatment of colonic cancer is by surgical resection of the colon with its draining lymph nodes. Carcinomas of the rectum can now be resected within 5 cm of the anal margin if the anastomosis is performed with a stapling device (low anterior resection). Different colonic operations are illustrated in Fig. 28.8.

Until recently radiotherapy and chemotherapy have had a limited role in the management of colorectal cancer, but many patients who have Dukes' C tumours now receive postoperative chemotherapy, which reduces recurrence rate by 40% and the mortality rate by 30%. A rectal cancer may be treated with preoperative radiotherapy.

Isolated liver metastases may be resected and 25% of cases survive 5 years.

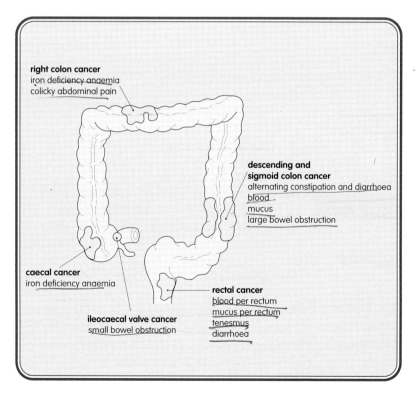

Fig. 28.7 Clinical presentations of colonic cancer. Approximately 70% of colonic cancers are in the left colon.

right colon cancer
iron deficiency anaemia
colicky abdominal pain

descending and sigmoid colon cancer
alternating constipation and diarrhoea
blood
mucus
large bowel obstruction

caecal cancer
iron deficiency anaemia

ileocaecal valve cancer
small bowel obstruction

rectal cancer
blood per rectum
mucus per rectum
tenesmus
diarrhoea

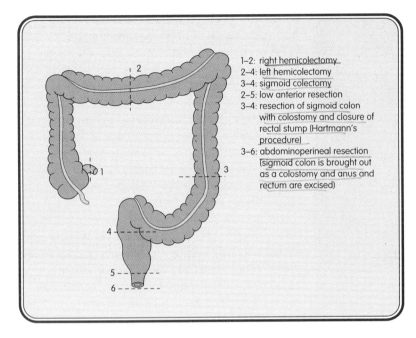

Fig. 28.8 Different types of colonic operation. Diagram to show the extent of the colonic resection for different operations.

1–2: right hemicolectomy
2–4: left hemicolectomy
3–4: sigmoid colectomy
2–5: low anterior resection
3–4: resection of sigmoid colon with colostomy and closure of rectal stump (Hartmann's procedure)
3–6: abdominoperineal resection (sigmoid colon is brought out as a colostomy and anus and rectum are excised)

VASCULAR DISORDERS

Angiodysplasia
Background
Angiodysplasia is a vascular abnormality that occurs in the elderly.

Clinical presentation
Angiodysplasia can cause spontaneous severe rectal bleeding. It usually occurs in the right colon and lesions are identified by arteriography if they are bleeding at a rate of 1–5 mL/min.

ISCHAEMIC COLITIS

Background
Ischaemic colitis occurs if there is atherosclerosis or increased blood viscosity.

Clinical presentation
The presenting symptom of ischaemic colitis is left-sided abdominal pain, which may be followed by bloody diarrhoea. It may be:
- Acute and cause gangrene and perforation.
- Chronic and cause a stricture, particularly at the splenic flexure of the colon.

COLONIC OBSTRUCTION

Background
Colonic obstruction is a common cause for an acute surgical admission.

Clinical presentation
The history of colonic obstruction is:
- Colicky abdominal pain.
- Abdominal distension.
- Increasing constipation progressing to absolute constipation.

There may be a preceding history of change of bowel habit. Vomiting may occur, but this is a late phenomenom. Causes of colonic obstruction are outlined in Fig. 28.9.

Management
Initial blood tests may show an iron deficiency anaemia suggesting an underlying colonic neoplasm. The patient may be dehydrated and have abnormal electrolytes. If the colon is perforated there will be free gas on an erect chest radiograph. An abdominal radiograph will show colonic dilatation with a 'cut-off' point. A limited barium enema (on unprepared bowel) is performed to confirm the level of the obstruction.

Causes of colonic obstruction	
Location	**Cause**
in the lumen	polypoid tumour, constipation
in the wall	malignant, ischaemic, diverticular or radiation stricture
outside colon	hernia, volvulus, intussusception

Fig. 28.9 Causes of colonic obstruction.

Before surgical intervention the patient is resuscitated. At laparotomy a colonic resection is performed. If the colon is obstructed and there is any associated sepsis it is not safe to perform an anastomosis so a colostomy is formed. The operations frequently performed are:

- Extended right hemicolectomy—for lesions of the ascending and transverse colon to the splenic flexure.
- Hartmann's procedure—resection of sigmoid colon, closure of rectal stump, and formation of an end-colostomy in the left iliac fossa.
- Subtotal colectomy—if the colon is grossly distended it may cause the caecum to perforate and then the whole of the colon is resected and an ileorectal anastomosis is formed.

- Double-barrelled colostomy—if there is a sigmoid volvulus (see Fig. 28.3) a sigmoid colectomy is performed and both ends are brought to the surface as a colostomy. This can be easily reversed without a second laparotomy.

Complications of a colostomy are:
- Retraction.
- Prolapse.
- Herniation.
- Stenosis.
- Bowel obstruction.

Colonic obstruction often occurs in the elderly population who have multiple medical problems and therefore the operation should be performed by experienced anaesthetists and surgeons to decrease the potential risks and any morbidity.

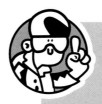

All patients who undergo emergency surgery for colonic problems should be warned that a colostomy may be necessary.

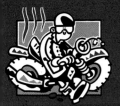

29. Anorectal Disorders

Anorectal problems are common and account for a large number of visits to general practitioners and referrals to surgical outpatient clinics. The common symptoms are:

- Rectal bleeding.
- Perianal swelling.
- Discomfort.
- Pruritus ani.

HAEMORRHOIDS

Background
A haemorrhoid is a venous plexus (anal cushion) that drains into the superior rectal vein accompanying the superior rectal artery. Haemorrhoids occupy the 3, 7, and 11 o'clock positions when looking at the anus in the lithotomy position. The venous plexuses become congested because:

- Straining increases the venous pressure.
- During pregnancy venous return is delayed by the presence of a pregnant uterus.

Clinical presentation
Symptoms of haemorrhoids are bright red rectal bleeding following defaecation, pruritus ani due to mucous discharge, and prolapse. The stages of 'piles' are outlined in Fig. 29.1.

If the haemorrhoids cannot be reduced it may be because the anal sphincter has gone into spasm and this is acutely painful and causes strangulation and thrombosis of the haemorrhoids.

Features of first-, second- and third-degree haemorrhoids	
Stage	**Appearance**
first degree	small and do not prolapse
second degree	small and prolapse, but reduce spontaneously
third degree	prolapsing 'piles' that have to be reduced manually

Fig. 29.1 Features of first-, second- and third-degree haemorrhoids.

Management
Haemorrhoids are diagnosed from the history and from examination of the anal canal with a proctoscope. General advice is given about a high-fibre diet to prevent constipation. First and second degree haemorrhoids can be treated by:

- Injection sclerotherapy—submucosal injection of phenol in almond oil into the base of the 'pile'. The injection is given using a proctoscope and should be painless because it is given above the dentate line.
- Barron's bands—rubber bands applied to the base of the haemorrhoid to constrict it so that it sloughs off 10 days later.
- Cryotherapy and infrared coagulation.
- Haemorrhoidectomy—if there is recurrent prolapse or the piles are acutely thrombosed. Each haemorrhoid is defined and its pedicle is transfixed and ligated. Complications of the operation include secondary haemorrhage at 10 days and anal stenosis.

ANAL FISSURE

Background
This is an acutely painful condition caused by straining, causing a superficial tear in the mucosa of the anal canal, usually posteriorly. There is secondary spasm of the external anal sphincter, which exacerbates the situation.

Clinical presentation
An anal fissure may cause some rectal bleeding. There is usually a history of throbbing severe perianal pain, which persists for some time after defaecation.

Management
On inspection the fissure will be visible with a sentinel 'pile' (skin tag). A rectal examination is often impossible due to spasm of the external anal sphincter.

Treatment options include the use of glyceryl trinitrate paste or local anaesthetic ointments together with an

Mory → strangulation + Thrombosis

anal dilator to overcome the sphincter spasm. If this does not relieve the situation a lateral external sphincterotomy is performed. This relieves the spasm and allows the sphincter to heal.

An anal stretch can be carried out, but there is a small risk of causing permanent sphincter damage resulting in partial incontinence.

PERIANAL HAEMATOMA

Background
Perianal haematoma is an acutely painful condition and results from rupture of a small blood vessel beneath the perianal skin.

Clinical presentation
Perianal haematoma presents as a bluish tender swelling that cannot be reduced. It is usually precipitated by constipation and straining.

Management
Most perianal haematomas resolve spontaneously in a few days. Alternatively the clot can be evacuated under local anaesthetic.

RECTAL PROLAPSE

Background
Rectal prolapse can occur in children, in whom it is a mucosal prolapse that resolves spontaneously.

A partial prolapse in adults can be treated with a submucosal injection of phenol, but in adults it is usually full thickness.

Important aetiological factors are:
- Chronic constipation.
- Multiparity in women, which may damage the pudendal nerves resulting in weakness of the sphincters.

Clinical presentation
Clinical presentations of rectal prolapse are:
- Discomfort of the prolapse, which may occur spontaneously or follow defaecation.
- Rectal bleeding.
- Mucus discharge.
- Incontinence.

Management
Treatment is usually surgical. If the patient is fit for a laparotomy a rectopexy is performed, which lifts the rectum and secures it to the hollow of the sacrum by a mesh or polytetrafluoroethylene sponge.

In elderly, frail patients local excision of the redundant rectal mucosa (Delorme's procedure) can be performed.

PERIANAL ABSCESS

Background
Perianal abscess is a very common problem requiring an acute surgical admission. The anal glands occur between the internal and external sphincters. A breach in the mucosa allows infection into the glands. This subsequently develops into an abscess, which then tracks inferiorly to the perianal region or laterally to the ischiorectal fossa where it can track to the opposite ischiorectal fossa (Fig. 29.2).

Clinical presentation
Patients present with a history of increasing discomfort in the perianal region with associated throbbing pain and swelling.

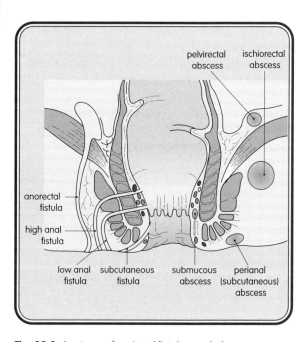

Fig. 29.2 Anatomy of perianal fistulae and abscesses.

Management

Inspection reveals a red, tender, inflamed, and indurated area, and the patient is pyrexial.

Treatment is by incision and drainage under general anaesthesia.

A swab is taken for bacteriology and if skin organisms such as staphylococci are grown the abscess is a simple skin infection, but if bowel organisms are grown there is possibly an underlying fistula.

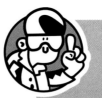

Goodsall's law—fistulae with external openings posterior to the meridian (East to West) in the lithotomy position usually open on the midline of the anus, whereas those with anterior external openings usually open directly into the anus.

If a perianal abscess contains bowel flora an underlying fistula should be suspected.

ANAL FISTULA

Background

A fistula is an abnormal communication between two epithelial surfaces (see Fig. 29.2). If a patient has recurrent infections in the same area or a persistent discharge then suspect a fistula. Perianal sepsis may also be associated with:

- Crohn's disease.
- Tuberculosis.
- Carcinoma of the rectum.

Management

Management consists of examination under anaesthetic. The external opening may be visible and it is probed to find the internal opening:

- If the internal opening is below the level of the internal sphincter the fistula track can be excised and left to granulate.
- If the fistula tracks above and through the sphincters a Seton suture is used (i.e. a nonabsorbable suture is passed along the fistula track). It is gradually tightened and causes a fibrous reaction as it cuts its way through the sphincter so there are no problems with incontinence.

Occasionally a defunctioning colostomy is formed before exploring a complex fistula.

Magnetic resonance imaging is a useful investigation for imaging a complex fistula.

PRURITUS ANI

Background

Pruritus ani may develop secondary to local causes in the rectum and anal canal causing mucus discharge. Common causes are:

- Haemorrhoids.
- Fistulae.
- Fungal infection.
- Thread worms.

Clinical presentation

Pruritus ani is irritation of the perianal skin.

Management

Treatment of pruritus ani comprises:

- Good hygiene.
- Treatment of the underlying cause.

ANAL CARCINOMA

Background

Anal carcinoma is a rare malignancy and usually occurs in elderly people. It is a squamous cell carcinoma that originates in the squamous mucosa of the lower anal canal. Rarer tumours include melanoma of the anal canal.

Most cases of squamous cell carcinoma arise *de novo*, but it may develop from an area of Bowen's disease (i.e. squamous carcinoma *in situ*) or it may be related to human papillomavirus infection (some women who have cervical intraepithelial neoplasia

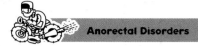

have similar changes in the mucosa of the vulva and anal canal).

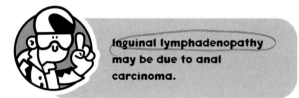

Inguinal lymphadenopathy may be due to anal carcinoma.

Clinical presentation

Presenting symptoms of anal carcinoma are:

- Perianal pain.
- Rectal bleeding.
- Discharge.
- Inguinal lymphadenopathy.

Management

A diagnosis of anal carcinoma is made by examination and biopsy.

Treatment is a combination of:

- Chemotherapy.
- Radiotherapy.
- Occasionally surgical excision of the rectum and anal canal by an abdominoperineal resection.

The prognosis of anal carcinoma is poor.

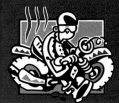

30. Hepatobiliary Disorders

NORMAL LIVER FUNCTION

The liver is the largest gland in the body and has two lobes and eight segments. Its functions include:
- Metabolism.
- Synthesis.
- Detoxification.
- Defence (see *Crash Course Gastrointestinal System* by E. Cheshire, Chapter 4).

The liver:
- Consumes approximately 20% of total body oxygen, and about 90% of the total hepatic blood flow is from the portal system.
- Produces about 600–1000 mL of bile per day and is responsible for secreting almost all of the body's bilirubin (i.e. a breakdown product of haem).
- Is an important site of hepatic protein synthesis and catabolism so albumin and protein levels are indicators of liver function.

ACUTE LIVER DAMAGE

Background
The liver can be damaged by a number of agents such as:
- Viruses (e.g. hepatitis A, B, or C).
- Drugs (e.g. alcohol, paracetamol).

Other causes of cirrhosis are cryptogenic or autoimmune (e.g. primary biliary cirrhosis) or secondary to biliary obstruction.

Management
Diagnosis of acute damage is based on the presence of high levels of serum transaminases and positive serology for hepatitis viruses.

Assessment of clotting function is another indicator of hepatic function because factors II, VII, IX, and X are manufactured in the liver with vitamin K.

Acute liver damage may progress to chronic liver damage, cirrhosis, portal hypertension, and liver failure.

Hepatitis serology should be checked for all patients who have jaundice of unknown cause.

PORTAL HYPERTENSION

Background
Portal hypertension develops if there is an elevated portal pressure of more than 15 mmHg, which can result from:
- Inflow or outflow obstruction.
- More rarely, increased portal blood flow in to the portal venous system due to an arteriovenous fistula between the portal vein and hepatic artery.

Causes of portal hypertension are:
- Prehepatic—portal vein thrombosis or occlusion by extrinsic compression.
- Intrahepatic—cirrhosis, periportal fibrosis, schistosomiasis.
- Posthepatic—veno-occlusive disease or Budd–Chiari syndrome.

Complications of portal hypertension
Portal hypertension is associated with the following complications:
- Splenomegaly—causes thrombocytopenia.
- Collateral circulation—demonstrated by the presence of oesophageal and gastric varices (which can bleed) or by caput medusae (i.e dilated veins around the umbilicus).
- Ascites—resulting from a low serum albumin concentration, increased aldosterone activity, and sodium retention, and increased portal pressure leading to transudation of fluid.

Remember that the causes of portal hypertension may be prehepatic, intrahepatic, or posthepatic.

- Resuscitation.
- Endoscopy and injection sclerotherapy.
- Tamponade with a Sengstaken–Blakemore tube (Fig. 30.1).
- Intravenous vasopressin or somatostatin—to lower the portal venous pressure.
- Surgical intervention by oesophageal transection or creating a portosystemic shunt.
- Transjugular intrahepatic portosystemic shunt —a new technique in which a stent is passed under radiological control from the internal jugular vein through the vena cava into the hepatic vein to create a shunt to decrease the pressure.

Management of bleeding oesophageal varices

The management of bleeding oesophageal varices may include:

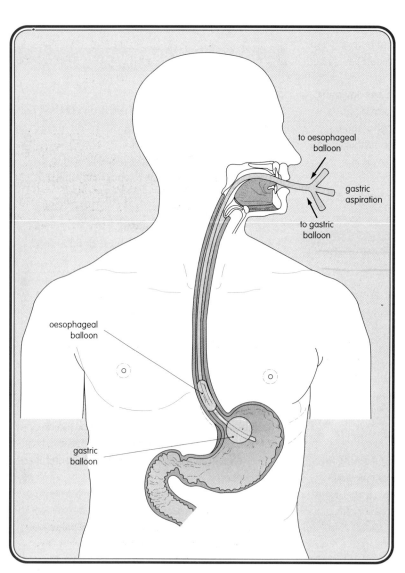

Fig. 30.1 A Sengstaken tube in position. It is used to control bleeding from oesophageal varices.

to oesophageal balloon

gastric aspiration

to gastric balloon

oesophageal balloon

gastric balloon

Risks from a variceal bleed

Patients who bleed from oesophageal varices already have an increased bleeding tendency because of impaired clotting and a decreased number of platelets. Hypovolaemia further damages liver function. Blood in the bowel is broken down by bacteria to release ammonia, which is absorbed and can cause hepatic encephalopathy. Oral lactulose and neomycin are used to reduce ammonia formation and absorption.

HEPATIC CYSTS

Background

The different groups of hepatic cysts are:
- Simple cysts—usually an incidental finding on ultrasound scan and asymptomatic.
- Cysts of polycystic disease—usually related to polycystic kidneys.
- Hydatid cysts—due to infection with *Echinococcus granulosus* or *Echinococcus multilocularis*. The infection is found in sheep and dogs and humans are the secondary host. It is endemic in sheep rearing areas. The cysts can become infected or rupture into the biliary tract or intraperitoneally. Treatment involves medication with mebendazole together with surgical excision.

HEPATIC ABSCESSES

Background

Hepatic abscesses can be intrahepatic or in the subphrenic or subhepatic spaces:
- Intrahepatic abscesses may be secondary to cholangitis or from spread of infection via the portal circulation from infections such as diverticulitis or appendicitis.
- Extrahepatic abscesses develop secondary to intra-abdominal sepsis.

Clinical presentation

The clinical features of hepatic abscesses are:
- Swinging pyrexia.
- Rigors.
- Jaundice.
- Vomiting.
- Right hypochondrial pain.
- Malaise.

Management

A diagnosis of hepatic abscess is made by an ultrasound scan, which is used to guide percutaneous drainage. This is combined with systemic antibiotics. Occasionally surgical drainage is required for multiloculated abscesses containing debris.

HEPATIC TUMOURS

Worldwide, primary hepatoma is a common cause of death, but in the UK most hepatic tumours are secondary tumours.

Primary benign hepatic tumours
Background
Primary benign hepatic tumours are rare, but include adenoma and focal nodular hyperplasia, which may be associated with use of the oral contraceptive.

Adenoma and focal nodular hyperplasia of the liver may be associated with oral contraceptive use.

Clinical presentation
Primary benign hepatic tumours may be asymptomatic, but they may cause pain and can rupture spontaneously and cause intraperitoneal bleeding.

Haemangiomas are common, but are usually asymptomatic.

Primary hepatoma
Background
Primary hepatoma can develop *de novo* in a cirrhotic liver. It is associated with hepatitis B infection and aflotoxins and is very common worldwide. Most cases present late.

Management
Diagnostic tests include the presence of elevated α-feto protein in the serum, ultrasound scan, and computed tomography (CT). Most tumours are not resectable and the prognosis is poor.

Cholangiocarcinoma
Background
Cholangiocarcinoma is a malignant tumour of the bile ducts.

Clinical presentation
Usually cholangiocarcinoma presents with painless obstructive jaundice.

Management
Cholangiocarcinoma is rarely resectable, but may be amenable to percutaneous or endoscopic stenting to give symptomatic relief.

Metastatic tumours
These are the commonest type of liver tumour. They are secondary deposits, particularly from:
- Breast.
- Colon.
- Stomach.
- Pancreas.
- Lung.
- Prostate.

Most are multiple and therefore not resectable.

Management
Palliative treatments can include systemic chemotherapy or via the hepatic artery, embolization, cryotherapy, or interstitial laser hyperthermia.

CHRONIC LIVER DISEASE

The clinical signs of chronic liver disease are shown in Fig. 30.2.

GALL BLADDER DISEASE

Most gall bladder problems are secondary to gall stones, which are very common. There may be a familial tendency and gall stones are more common in females than males. Other predisposing factors are:
- Obesity.
- Multiparity.
- Chronic haemolytic disease.
- Ileal disease or resection.

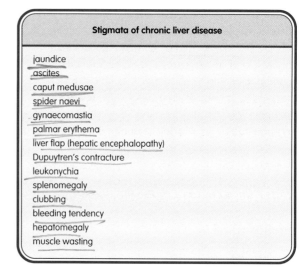

Stigmata of chronic liver disease
jaundice
ascites
caput medusae
spider naevi
gynaecomastia
palmar erythema
liver flap (hepatic encephalopathy)
Dupuytren's contracture
leukonychia
splenomegaly
clubbing
bleeding tendency
hepatomegaly
muscle wasting

Fig. 30.2 Stigmata of chronic liver disease.

- Drugs such as oral contraceptives, diuretics, and clofibrate.

Gall stones are formed of cholesterol or bile pigments or are mixed stones.

Pathogenesis of gall stones
Cholesterol stones
Normally cholesterol and phospholipids are held in solution by being surrounded by bile salts. When there is an imbalance cholesterol crystals form and lead to the formation of stones.

Bilirubin and pigment stones
These may occur in patients who have chronic haemolytic disorders in which there is excessive production of bile pigments.

Alternatively certain bacteria contain an enzyme, glucuronidase, which splits bilirubin and then combines with calcium to form calcium bilirubinate.

Over 90% of gallstones are not calcified and so do not show up on a plain abdominal radiograph.

Clinical presentation

Problems from gall stones are often triggered by ingestion of fatty food because it stimulates the production of cholecystokinin, which stimulates the gall bladder to contract to release bile to digest the fat.

The clinical presentation of gall stones may be:

- Asymptomatic—an incidental finding on ultrasound.
- Biliary colic—a severe episode of pain in the right hypochondrium that radiates to the tip of the scapula. Pain makes the patient restless and may last several hours and be associated with vomiting and sweating. Biliary colic is due to a gall stone temporarily obstructing the cystic duct or Hartmann's pouch.
- Acute cholecystitis—this may be preceded by biliary colic, but then the pain becomes localized and persistent in the right hypochondrium. It is associated with vomiting and on examination the patient will have a pyrexia and a positive Murphy's sign. It is due to chemical inflammation and secondary bacterial infection of an obstructed gall bladder. It may resolve with antibiotics for Gram-negative organisms.
- Mucocele—this forms if the gall bladder remains obstructed and the contents are sterile.
- Empyema—this forms if the gall bladder is obstructed and infection persists despite antibiotics.
- Perforated gall bladder—this occurs if the obstructed gall bladder becomes overdistended and the fundus is ischaemic so that peritonitis develops.
- Gall bladder fistula—an inflamed gall bladder may become adherent to adjacent structures such as the duodenum. Persistent inflammation may cause a fistula to develop between the structures so that a large gall stone can pass into the small intestine and present with small bowel obstruction, (i.e. gall stone ileus).
- Chronic cholecystitis—the gall bladder is thick walled and shrunken. The symptoms are chronic and non-specific, such as upper abdominal discomfort, flatulence, fatty food intolerance, epigastric or right hypochondrial pain, and nausea.

Complications of gall stones

Gall stones may pass from the gall bladder into the common bile duct and cause several problems (Fig. 30.3), including:

- Pancreatitis—a stone may temporarily obstruct the pancreatic duct and cause pancreatic inflammation.
- Obstructive jaundice—a stone may lodge in the common bile duct, preventing the drainage of bile so the patient has symptoms and signs of obstructive jaundice.
- Ascending cholangitis—if infection develops in an obstructed biliary system the patient is seriously ill with fever, rigors, and jaundice (Charcot's triad), and is at risk of developing septicaemia.

An uncommon complication of chronic gall stone disease is the development of carcinoma of the gall bladder. It is usually discovered late when it has already invaded adjacent structures so the prognosis is poor. Occasionally carcinoma of the gall bladder is an incidental finding after cholecystectomy.

Pathologically 90% of gall bladder carcinomas are adenocarcinomas and 10% are squamous cell carcinomas.

Management

Gall stones are usually diagnosed by ultrasound scan. Management plans are as follows:

- Asymptomatic—no treatment required.
- Chronic cholecystitis—patients are given advice about a low-fat diet and advised to have a cholecystectomy, which is usually performed laparoscopically. Patients should always be warned that it may be necessary to convert to an open cholecystectomy if it is not possible to perform a safe operation due to gross inflammation or technical difficulties.
- Acute cholecystitis—patients are treated with analgesia, intravenous fluids, and antibiotics. If this does not resolve cholecystectomy is required urgently, otherwise it is performed at a later date.
- Perforated gall bladder—peritonitis requires an emergency laparotomy and cholecystectomy.
- Empyema—if the patient is fit for an operation a cholecystectomy is performed, but if the patient is unfit a cholecystostomy (i.e. percutaneous drainage of the abscess) can be performed instead.
- Gall stone ileus—this is usually diagnosed during a laparotomy for small bowel obstruction. The diagnosis may be suspected if a preoperative abdominal radiograph shows gas in the biliary tree. The gall stone is removed from the ileum by an enterotomy, but the choleduodenal fistula is left because it will seal spontaneously.

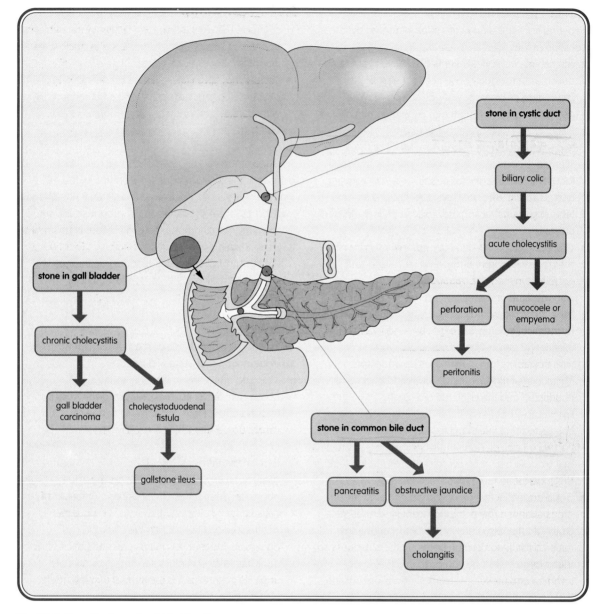

Fig. 30.3 Complications of gall bladder disease.

- Common bile duct stones—patients are jaundiced clinically and biochemically. The ultrasound scan will show a dilated bile duct and urgent endoscopic retrograde cholangiopancreatography (ERCP) is performed to remove the stones so the bile can drain freely to decrease the risk from infection. If there are signs of cholangitis the patient is also treated with intravenous fluids and antibiotics.

Some patients are not fit for surgical treatment or decline an operation. Non-surgical treatments are available, but are not very effective and have marked side effects. For the treatments to be effective:

- The gall bladder needs to be capable of contractions.
- The stones should be radiolucent and less than 15 mm in diameter.

Non-surgical treatments include the use of extracorporeal shock wave lithotripsy. This shatters the stones into small pieces, which are then passed out of the gall bladder, but the patients also have to ingest bile salts such as chenodeoxycholic acid to prevent the stones from reforming.

ACALCULOUS CHOLECYSTITIS

Background

Acalculous cholecystitis is a rare problem, but occurs in seriously ill patients who are already requiring intensive treatment (e.g. following cardiac surgery, multiple trauma, or burns). Acute inflammation of the gall bladder may result from stasis and secondary infection. Cholecystectomy may be required.

Other acalculous conditions are:
- Cholesterolosis (strawberry gall bladder, i.e. cholesterol deposits in the gall bladder wall).
- Adenomyomatosis (cholecystitis glandularis proliferans).
- Porcelain gall bladder (calcification of the gall bladder).

PANCREATITIS

Background

This is an acute inflammatory condition of the exocrine pancreas. Acinar injury occurs, releasing pancreatic enzymes into the circulation and the peritoneal cavity. It can be a mild disease or very severe with life-threatening complications.

Common causes are:
- Duct obstruction—due to gall stones, tumours, abnormal anatomy of the pancreas.
- Acinar cell injury—due to alcohol, steroids, diuretics, hypothermia, hypercalcaemia, hyperlipidaemia, viruses (eg. coxsackievirus and mumps), or trauma.

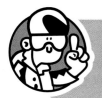

Gall stones and alcohol cause 95% of cases of pancreatitis.

Clinical presentation

Patients present with an acute onset of severe constant epigastric pain, which often radiates to the back. There may be associated symptoms of nausea or vomiting. The history may give clues about the likely aetiology. Clinical signs may include:
- Tachycardia.
- Hypotension.
- Pyrexia.
- Jaundice.
- Upper abdominal tenderness.
- Peritonism.

If the symptoms have been present for a few days there may be bruising of the abdominal wall due to tracking of a blood-stained exudate:
- Grey Turner's sign in the flank.
- Cullen's sign in the periumbilical region.

If the patient is developing severe necrotizing pancreatitis there may be signs of:
- Hypotension due to septicaemia.
- Respiratory depression.
- Diffuse abdominal tenderness with distension because of ascites.
- Absent bowel sounds due to an ileus.

Management

Effective management of pancreatitis is by:
- Diagnosis—this is made by detecting an elevated serum amylase (i.e. >1000 IU/mL). An abdominal radiograph may show a sentinel loop of small intestine in the region of the pancreas. The important differential diagnosis is a perforated peptic ulcer and this diagnosis is confirmed by the presence of free subdiaphragmatic gas on an erect chest radiograph. Other investigations are performed to assess the severity of the condition according to the Imrie–Ransom criteria (Fig. 30.4).
- Resuscitation—intravenous fluids, oxygenation.
- Intensive monitoring—pulse, blood pressure, oxygen saturation, temperature, renal function, glucose, and calcium levels.
- Analgesia.
- Imaging of pancreas—an ultrasound is useful to diagnose gall stones and pancreatic pseudocysts, but if the patient has severe haemorrhagic or

Investigations to assess the severity of pancreatitis	
Type of investigation	**Parameter**
clinical	hypotension
	respiratory difficulty
laboratory	white cell count >16 × 10⁹/L
	Po_2 <7.98 kPa (60 mmHg)
	blood glucose >11.2 mmol/L
	serum lactate dehydrogenase (LDH) >350 IU/L
	aspartate transaminase (AST) (also known as serum glutamic-oxaloacetic transaminase, SGOT) >250 IU/L
	packed cell volume (PCV) ↓ >10%
	blood urea >18 mmol/L
	serum calcium <2.0 mmol/L

Fig. 30.4 Investigations to assess the severity of pancreatitis (Imrie–Ransom criteria).

necrotizing pancreatitis a CT scan is essential to assess the extent of necrotic tissue, which may require surgical debridement.

- ERCP—this is performed to clear the bile duct of any gall stones if this is the cause.
- Cholecystectomy—if the pancreatitis is caused by gall stones a cholecystectomy is necessary to prevent further episodes.

Other causes should be treated appropriately (e.g. complete abstinence from alcohol).

Complications of acute pancreatitis
Complications that can be associated with acute pancreatitis are:

- Pancreatic pseudocyst—this may follow mild or moderate pancreatitis. It is a collection of fluid in the lesser sac (i.e. between the stomach and the pancreas). It may be asymptomatic or cause gastric compression or an abdominal swelling. It is diagnosed by ultrasound scan. If small it may resolve or it can be drained percutaneously. Large or recurrent cysts require surgical drainage into the

stomach (i.e. cystgastrostomy) or into the small intestine.

- Pancreatic necrosis, abscess, or intra-abdominal sepsis—these follow severe pancreatitis. They are diagnosed by CT scan and the poor condition of the patient. Urgent laparotomy with radical operative debridement of necrotic tissue is required. The patient requires intensive monitoring in the intensive care unit.
- Pancreatic haemorrhage.
- Acute respiratory distress syndrome.
- Renal failure.

CHRONIC PANCREATITIS

Background
Recurrent episodes of acute pancreatitis cause permanent damage to the pancreas, which becomes fibrotic and unable to fulfil its exocrine or endocrine functions. The commonest cause is alcohol abuse.

Clinical presentation
The symptoms of chronic pancreatitis are chronic severe epigastric and back pain associated with the development of steatorrhoea, malnutrition, and diabetes mellitus. Other presentations may include obstructive jaundice or duodenal obstruction, which may require treatment with a bypass procedure.

Management
Treatment of chronic pancreatitis is aimed at controlling symptoms and comprises:
- Strong analgesics.
- Pancreatic enzyme supplements.
- Diabetic regimens.

Pancreatectomy is occasionally performed.

PANCREATIC TUMOURS

Background
These can arise from the exocrine or endocrine cells of the pancreas. The commonest tumour is an

adenocarcinoma of the pancreas. The incidence of pancreatic carcinoma is increasing and it usually occurs in people over 50 years of age. Predisposing factors may include alcohol, diabetes mellitus, and chronic pancreatitis.

Clnical presentation

Most pancreatic tumours present late with symptoms such as:
- Obstructive jaundice if the head of the pancreas is involved.
- Vomiting if there is duodenal obstruction.
- Severe intractable back pain if the body and tail are involved.
- Unexplained weight loss.

Occasionally a small periampullary tumour presents early with obstructive jaundice.

Management

Effective management is by:
- Diagnosis—based on clinical suspicion. An ultrasound scan may show a dilated biliary tree and pancreatic mass. A CT scan will provide more accurate information about the extent of tumour and operability. An ERCP may demonstrate a periampullary tumour and enable biopsies to be taken from it or brush cytology from the pancreas. Tumour markers such as CA19-9 allow disease progress to be assessed.
- Treatment—most patients present late when the tumour is inoperable so treatment is palliative in the form of analgesia, insertion of a stent to relieve obstructive jaundice or gastroenterostomy for duodenal obstruction.

The prognosis is poor and 90% of patients die within 1 year.

Periampullary tumours may be small and resectable by a pancreaticoduodenectomy (i.e. resection of head of pancreas, duodenum, and common bile duct). The prognosis of these tumours is better and 50% of patients are alive at 5 years.

ENDOCRINE TUMOURS OF THE PANCREAS

Background

Endocrine tumours of the pancreas are uncommon, but are detected by the recognition of clinical syndromes.

Management

A diagnosis of endocrine tumour of the pancreas is made by the detection of abnormal serum hormone levels by radioimmunoassay. The tumours are localized and staged by CT scans.

The commonest tumour is an insulinoma and 90% of these are benign and solitary so they should be surgically resected. The other tumours are more likely to be malignant and may only be suitable for symptomatic treatment.

Fig. 30.5 summarizes the different types of endocrine tumours and their clinical effects.

Endocrine tumours of pancreas		
Tumour	Hormone secreted	Effects
insulinoma	insulin	hypoglycaemia
gastrinoma	gastrin	Zollinger–Ellison syndrome, intractable peptic ulceration
glucagonoma	glucagon	diabetes mellitus, necrotic migratory erythema, weight loss, weakness, stomatitis
somatostatinoma	somatostatin	diabetes mellitus, gall stones, malabsorption

Fig. 30.5 Endocrine tumours of the pancreas.

Causes of obstructive jaundice	
Location	Cause
in the lumen of the bile duct	gallstones *Clonorchis sinensis* (liver fluke)
in the wall of the bile duct	cholangiocarcinoma benign strictures sclerosing cholangitis carcinoma of ampulla of Vater
outside the bile duct	porta hepatis nodes pancreatic cancer gall bladder cancer chronic pancreatitis

Fig. 30.6 Causes of obstructive jaundice.

OBSTRUCTIVE JAUNDICE

Clinical presentation

A diagnosis of obstructive jaundice is based upon a clinical history of jaundice, pale stools, dark urine, and pruritus, with or without pain.

Management

Investigations include:
- Full blood count.
- Clotting screen. + PT + Albumin
- Urea and electrolytes—for baseline renal function.
- Liver function tests—show increased bilirubin, alkaline phosphatase, and γ-glutamyltransferase.
- Ultrasound scan—shows a dilated biliary tree and may reveal the cause (e.g. gall stones or pancreatic tumour).
- ERCP—can be used to define the level of the obstruction, take biopsies, remove gall stones, or insert a stent.
- Percutaneous transhepatic cholangiography—can be used to define the level of obstruction if unable to do an ERCP and a stent can also be inserted percutaneously to bypass an obstruction.

- CT scan—can be used to stage and assess operability of a tumour.

The causes of obstructive jaundice are given in Fig. 30.6.

Complications of obstructive jaundice

Before any invasive procedure, either radiological or surgical, precautions should be taken to prevent complications of obstructive jaundice such as:
- Cholangitis—infection manifested as rigors, pyrexia, and hypotension.
- Renal failure—this may be precipitated by septicaemia or may be due to the absorption of endotoxins from the bowel and their reduced hepatic clearance. Endotoxins can cause acute tubular necrosis and peritubular fibrin deposition.
- Disseminated intravascular coagulation.
- Delayed wound healing and gastrointestinal haemorrhage.

To prevent these complications patients should be resuscitated and well hydrated to maintain renal perfusion. Abnormal clotting is corrected by administering vitamin K and other clotting factors. Administration of oral lactulose decreases the risk of endotoxaemia. Any infection is treated and prophylactic intravenous antibiotics are given before an invasive procedure.

The treatment of jaundice is:
- Use of a stent for inoperable malignant tumours.
- Removal of gallstones by ERCP or open surgery of the bile duct.

Fig. 30.7 illustrates Courvoisier's Law, which states that in the presence of jaundice if the gall bladder is palpable then the jaundice is unlikely to be due to a stone because the gall bladder is usually shrunken and fibrotic with gall stones. The exception to this rule is a stone stuck in Hartmann's pouch with another stone in the common bile duct.

Fig. 30.7 Courvoisier's law.

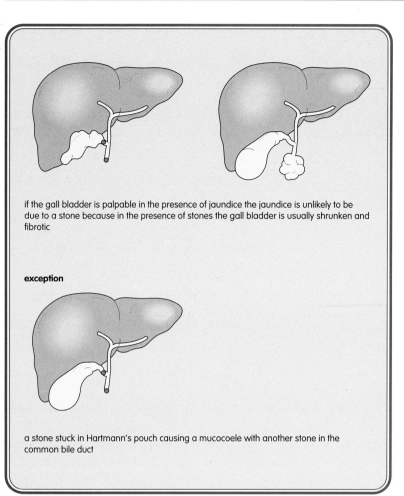

if the gall bladder is palpable in the presence of jaundice the jaundice is unlikely to be due to a stone because in the presence of stones the gall bladder is usually shrunken and fibrotic

exception

a stone stuck in Hartmann's pouch causing a mucocoele with another stone in the common bile duct

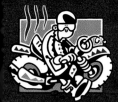

31. Gynaecological Disorders

Women who present with lower abdominal pain may have a gynaecological problem. It is usually a benign condition and may be part of the normal menstrual cycle (e.g. mittelschmerz pain or midcycle pain) due to ovulation. Another common cause of pain is dysmenorrhoea (i.e. pain due to menstruation) and this can be of variable severity. It may be associated with:

- Excessive uterine contractions.
- Endometriosis.
- Pelvic inflammatory disease.

Other symptoms may be menorrhagia, dyspareunia, or infertility.

OVARIAN CYSTS AND NEOPLASMS

Many cysts are asymptomatic and are detected by pelvic ultrasound. The different benign cysts are:

- Follicular cysts—simple thin-walled cysts, which are asymptomatic and resolve spontaneously.
- Corpus luteum cyst—forms after ovulation.
- Endometriosis cyst—this is due to bleeding into a deposit of endometriosis and the blood becomes thick and tarry to form a 'chocolate cyst'.

OVARIAN TUMOURS

Background
Ovarian tumours usually have solid and cystic elements. They are classified as benign or malignant, and serous or mucinous or endometroid tumours.

An unusual type of benign tumour is a teratoma or dermoid cyst, which usually occurs in women aged between 20 and 30 years, and 20% are bilateral. It is a cystic tumour and may contain a variety of structures such as hair, teeth, skin, or cartilage.

Ovarian cancer often presents with vague symptoms and is initially painless.

Clinical presentation
Ovarian tumours may be asymptomatic or they may present with abdominal distension from a large benign cyst or from ascites if the tumour is malignant. Pressure symptoms may cause frequency of micturition. Abdominal pain is a symptom if a complication occurs.

If the tumour is malignant there may be systemic features of malignancy such as weight loss.

Complications
Complications associated with ovarian cysts and tumours are:

- Torsion—this causes severe lower abdominal pain with vomiting. There may be a history of preceding episodes that resolved.
- Rupture—if the cyst is small and benign it is probably asymptomatic. If a malignant tumour ruptures this causes severe lower abdominal pain with vomiting and circulatory collapse.
- Haemorrhage into a cyst—this causes similar symptoms to torsion.

Management
Diagnosis is usually made by pelvic ultrasound. If a complication has occurred to a benign cyst or tumour then laparoscopic or open surgical intervention is required.

If malignancy is suspected, the tumour marker CA125 may be elevated and computed tomography can be used to assess stage and operability:

- If operable, bilateral oophorectomies, a hysterectomy, and omentectomy are performed.

- If technically inoperable due to widespread intraperitoneal disease, the tumour is debulked as much as possible and any residual disease is treated with chemotherapy, which has dramatically improved the prognosis of ovarian cancer.

PELVIC INFLAMMATORY DISEASE

Background

Pelvic inflammatory disease can be an acute condition or have a more chronic course. Infection may follow delivery or abortion or commonly it is sexually transmitted. The causative organisms are:

- *Streptococcus* or *Staphylococcus* spp. after operative intervention.
- *Neisseria gonorrhoeae* and *Chlamydia trachomatis* are implicated in sexually transmitted infection.

Clinical presentation

The symptoms of acute infection are:

- Lower abdominal pain.
- Dyspareunia.
- Vaginal discharge.
- Malaise.
- Fever.

Management

Clinical examination will produce tenderness of the lower abdomen and on vaginal examination. A high vaginal swab is taken to find the causative organism. A pelvic ultrasound is carried out to look for complications (Fig. 31.1) such as:

- Hydrosalpinx—an obstructed swollen fallopian tube.
- Pyosalpinx—an obstructed fallopian tube containing pus.
- Tuboovarian abscess—an inflammatory process involving the fallopian tube and ovary, which may rupture to cause peritonitis.

Most cases of pelvic inflammatory disease are managed conservatively with analgesia and appropriate antibiotics. Surgical intervention is required for a complication suggesting ongoing sepsis.

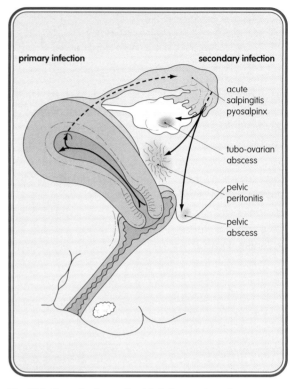

Fig. 31.1 Complications of pelvic inflammatory disease.

Some patients develop chronic pelvic inflammatory disease due to subacute recurrent infections. This causes chronic pelvic pain, dyspareunia, infertility, and an increased risk of an ectopic pregnancy.

ECTOPIC PREGNANCY

Background

A diagnosis of pregnancy should be excluded in all women of reproductive age who present with lower abdominal pain in case they have an ectopic pregnancy. This is a fertilized ovum, which implants outside the uterus, usually in the fallopian tube.

Predisposing factors are pelvic inflammatory disease and the presence of an intrauterine contraceptive device.

Pregnancy should be excluded in young women who have lower abdominal pain because of the risk of an ectopic pregnancy.

Clinical presentation

The symptoms of ectopic pregnancy occur about 6–8 weeks after conception. There is usually a history of a missed period and possibly a positive pregnancy test. The patient will complain of lower abdominal pain, which is due to distension of the fallopian tube, and there may be some vaginal bleeding.

If the pain becomes more severe and there is circulatory collapse the pregnancy has ruptured into the peritoneal cavity.

Management

The diagnosis is made from the history, together with a positive pregnancy test and an ultrasound scan, which demonstrates the swollen tube.

If the patient presents with acute collapse an emergency laparotomy is required.

All ectopic pregnancies have to be removed either laparoscopically or at open surgery to prevent rupture. If possible efforts are made to preserve the fallopian tube.

ENDOMETRIOSIS

Background

Endometriosis is a common uterine disorder and is due to ectopic deposits of endometrial cells in the lower part of the peritoneal cavity.

Clinical presentation

The main symptom of endometriosis is premenstrual pain that reaches a peak during menstruation and then gradually subsides.

Management

Endometriosis is treated by suppressing ovarian function.

LEIOMYOMA

Leiomyoma is a benign tumour of the myometrium.

Most fibroids are asymptomatic, but they may cause menorrhagia. Pelvic pain may occur if a pedunculated submucous fibroid undergoes torsion or infarcts during pregnancy.

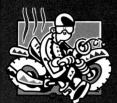

32. Abdominal Hernias

A hernia is a protrusion of a viscus or part of a viscus through its covering into an abnormal situation. A hernia consists of :

- Contents.
- Sac (e.g. peritoneum).
- External coverings.

Hernias occur at natural points of weakness (e.g. umbilicus, inguinal canal or femoral canal; Fig. 32.1), but may be caused by nerve damage causing muscle weakness. Such weaknesses may be exacerbated by conditions that increase intra-abdominal pressure such as ascites, chronic cough, constipation, urinary outflow obstruction, and heavy lifting.

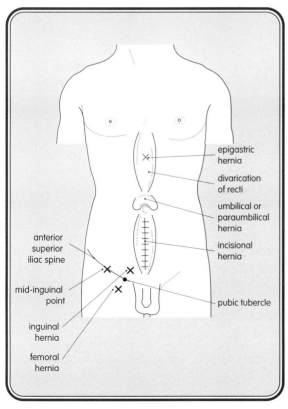

Fig. 32.1 Hernia sites.

(Figure labels: epigastric hernia, divarication of recti, umbilical or paraumbilical hernia, incisional hernia, anterior superior iliac spine, mid-inguinal point, inguinal hernia, femoral hernia, pubic tubercle)

TYPES OF HERNIA

The four major types of hernia illustrated in Fig. 32.2 are:

- Reducible—the contents of the hernia will return easily to the peritoneal cavity.
- Irreducible—adhesions form between the contents and the sac so it is impossible to reduce the bowel or omentum, but is viable.
- Strangulated—the contents of the sac become stuck through the hernial orifice and the blood supply is cut off so the bowel becomes ischaemic. Patients have symptoms of small bowel obstruction and the hernia is a tender inflamed swelling.
- Sliding—the sac may contain bowel, which is adherent to the sac so it cannot be reduced separately (e.g. sigmoid colon).

Hernias with narrow necks have a high risk of strangulation. The frequency of strangulation for different types of hernia in descending order is:
- Femoral
- Indirect inguinal
- Paraumbilical

INGUINAL HERNIA

Background

The anatomy of the inguinal canal and the two different types of inguinal hernia (direct and indirect hernias) is shown in Fig. 32.3.

- Indirect inguinal hernia may be congenital due to failure of obliteration of the processus vaginalis. It can also be acquired later in life when the sac emerges through the deep ring and passes along the inguinal canal together with the vas deferens and

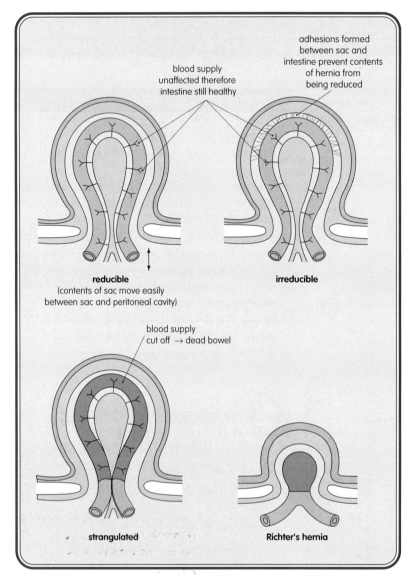

Fig. 32.2 Types of hernia.

acquires the coverings of the cord. It may emerge through the superficial ring into the upper scrotum.

- Direct inguinal hernia occurs as a result of weakness in the transversalis fascia in Hasselbach's triangle.

Management

Inguinal hernias should be repaired, especially if indirect. In children a herniotomy (i.e. excision of the sac) is sufficient, but in adults a herniotomy is accompanied by repair of the weakness in the posterior wall of the inguinal canal. This can be done using a non-absorbable suture darn technique, but this is being superseded by the use of a non-absorbable synthetic mesh, which is used to produce a non-tension repair (Lichenstein technique). This has the lowest risk of recurrence because it does not rely on the strength of the tissues.

A truss is of no significant benefit and many patients can have a hernia repaired under regional anaesthesia rather than a general anaesthetic.

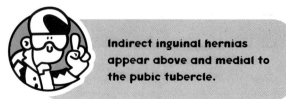

Indirect inguinal hernias appear above and medial to the pubic tubercle.

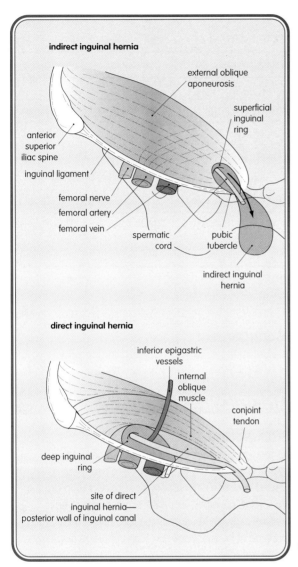

Fig. 32.3 Anatomy of the inguinal canal to demonstrate indirect and direct inguinal hernias.

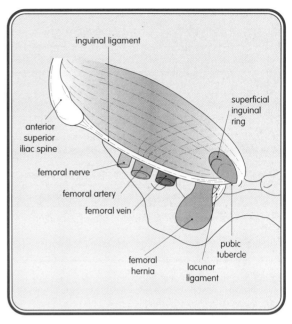

Fig. 32.4 Anatomy of a femoral hernia.

If the hernia contains small intestine it may be necessary to extend the incision to allow access to the peritoneal cavity to resect the bowel.

Fig. 32.5 compares the features of indirect and direct inguinal hernias, and femoral hernias.

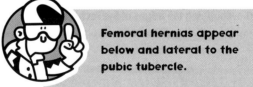

Femoral hernias appear below and lateral to the pubic tubercle.

FEMORAL HERNIA

The anatomy of a femoral hernia is shown in Fig. 32.4.

Management

All femoral hernias should be repaired because of the high risk of strangulation. There are several surgical approaches to a femoral hernia—low or high or via the posterior aspect of the inguinal canal. The sac is identified, the contents reduced, and the femoral canal obliterated with nonabsorbable sutures.

UMBILICAL HERNIA

Background

An umbilical hernia results from a congenital weakness due to persistence of an abdominal wall defect at the site of the umbilicus.

Management

Most umbilical hernias close spontaneously and an operation should not be performed until the child is at least 2 years old unless it becomes irreducible and strangulates.

Comparison of inguinal and femoral hernias			
Feature	Indirect inguinal	Direct inguinal	Femoral
Sex	m>f	m>f	f>m
Pathogenesis	may be congenital or acquired	acquired	acquired
Age	children, adults	adults	>middle aged
Descent into scrotum	may descend to scrotum	no	no
Reduction	does not reduce immediately	spontaneously on lying down	does not reduce spontaneously
Relationship to pubic tubercle	above and medial	above and lateral	below and lateral
Controlled by pressure over deep ring	yes	no	no
Risk of strangulation	high	very rare	high

Fig. 32.5 Comparison of inguinal and femoral hernias.

PARAUMBILICAL HERNIA

Background
A paraumbilical hernia results from an acquired weakness, especially in obese adults. The defect is just above the umbilicus. The sac often contains omentum or small intestine.

Management
A paraumbilical hernia has a marked risk of strangulation so it should be repaired by excising the sac and overlapping the edges of the rectus sheath (Mayo repair) with non-absorbable sutures.

EPIGASTRIC HERNIA

Background
An epigastric hernia is a small defect in the linea alba between the xiphisternum and the umbilicus, which usually contains only extraperitoneal fat, but can be very painful. It does not usually have a sac.

An epigastric hernia can cause marked epigastric pain, mimicking that of a peptic ulcer.

Management
The defect is closed with non-absorbable sutures.

INCISIONAL HERNIA

Background
An incisional hernia occurs through a defect in a scar. It is more likely to occur if there has been a wound infection or haematoma. Patients who are jaundiced, cachexic, or on corticosteroids, or have a chronic cough have an increased risk of developing this type of hernia. Poor surgical technique also plays a marked role.

Management
Although the defect resulting in an incisional hernia is often large and the risk of strangulation is low the appearance is unsightly and most patients want the hernia to be repaired. This may be done with sutures if the muscle is strong enough or it may need repair with a synthetic mesh.

UNCOMMON HERNIAS

Richter's hernia
This is an uncommon hernia and is a variant of a strangulated hernia in which only part of the bowel wall is strangulated.

The patient will have some symptoms of abdominal pain and vomiting, but not absolute constipation. The diagnosis may therefore be delayed until the bowel perforates into the hernia sac.

Spigelian hernia

This very rare hernia occurs through the defect at the lateral border of the rectus abdominis muscle after emerging through a defect in the transversus and internal oblique fascia halfway between the umbilicus and the pubic symphysis.

Gluteal hernia

This type of hernia crosses the greater sciatic notch

Sciatic hernia

A sciatic hernia passes through the lesser sciatic notch

Lumbar hernia

A lumbar hernia passes through the inferior lumbar triangle bounded by the iliac crest, the latissimus dorsi medially, and the external oblique laterally.

DIAPHRAGMATIC HERNIA

Background

A diaphragmatic hernia is an internal hernia and may be a congenital defect, which may be evident soon after birth.

The other cause of a diaphragmatic hernia is trauma. The left diaphragm is more commonly injured than the right. Minor tears may not be immediately apparent, but may present several years later with an incarcerated diaphragmatic hernia (i.e. with symptoms of bowel obstruction).

Clinical presentation

The newborn baby has breathing difficulties because the left side of the chest is occupied by the bowel rather than the lung. This is due to incomplete fusion of parts of the diaphragm.

Management

A diaphragmatic hernia requires urgent surgical repair.

OBTURATOR HERNIA

Background

This internal hernia occurs in frail elderly women.

Clinical presentation

The hernia occurs through the obturator canal within the pelvis, so the patient presents with small bowel obstruction. There may be pain along the medial aspect of the thigh because of pressure on the obturator nerve causing referred pain in its area of cutaneous distribution.

Management

Obturator hernia is rare and is usually only diagnosed at laparotomy for obstruction

RECTUS HAEMATOMA

This abdominal wall swelling develops after abdominal wall straining (e.g. coughing or lifting) and is due to tearing of branches of the inferior epigastric artery. It is common in elderly patients who are being treated with anticoagulants.

Clinical presentation

Rectus haematoma causes severe localized lower abdominal wall pain with a tender mass related to the lower part of the rectus sheath.

Management

A diagnosis of rectus haematoma may be confirmed by an ultrasound scan and in most cases it is managed conservatively by analgesia and correcting any coagulation problem.

DESMOID TUMOUR

This is a slow-growing tumour of the rectus abdominis muscle that usually occurs in young people. It may be related to Gardner's syndrome and may follow pregnancy. It is a tumour of spindle cells and there is a risk of local recurrence after excision.

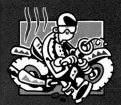

33. Thyroid and Parathyroid Disorders

THYROID GLAND

The thyroid gland develops from an endodermal outgrowth from the floor of the pharynx, which subsequently becomes the foramen caecum at the junction of the anterior two-thirds and the posterior one-third of the tongue. The tissue migrates towards the suprasternal notch. Below the larynx it becomes a bilobed structure and it proliferates to form the glandular tissue. The thyroglossal duct atrophies, but remnants may persist to become cysts. Ectopic thyroid tissue may be found anywhere along the route of the thyroid gland.

Physiology

The thyroid gland is responsible for synthesizing thyroid hormones:

- Thyroxine (T_4).
- Tri-iodothyronine (T_3).

These are responsible for maintaining normal metabolism. The gland can become under- or overactive for a number of different reasons, resulting in a range of abnormal symptoms. Tri-iodothyronine and T_4 secretion are controlled by the hypothalamus and the anterior pituitary gland, which releases thyroid stimulating hormone (TSH).

THYROGLOSSAL CYST

Background

A thyroglossal cyst is a midline swelling of the neck (see Chapter 34, Fig. 34.2). It is usually located below the hyoid bone and because it is connected to the base of the tongue it moves up on swallowing and when the tongue is protruded. The cyst may become infected or discharge.

Management

Treatment of a thyroglossal cyst is by surgical excision. The cyst is excised together with its fibrous tract extending to the foramen caecum, and it is often necessary to excise the hyoid bone.

Infection of a cyst or incomplete excision may produce a fistula track, discharging pus.

THYROID GOITRE

Background

Thyroid goitre is an abnormal swelling of the thyroid gland. Patients who have a goitre can be euthyroid, hypothyroid, or hyperthyroid (Fig. 33.1).

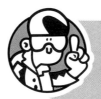

Secondary thyrotoxicosis causes predominantly cardiovascular symptoms.

Causes of goitre include:

- Normal physiological change—for example in puberty or during pregnancy.
- Iodine deficiency—a dietary deficiency of iodine results in increased TSH activity to stimulate the gland to produce enough thyroxine, so the gland enlarges.
- Graves' disease—a diffuse smooth vascular swelling of the thyroid gland associated with thyrotoxicosis and eye problems such as exophthalmos, lid lag, and ophthalmoplegia. Graves' disease is due to the presence of long-acting thyroid stimulating immunoglobulin (LATS).
- Benign hyperplasia of the thyroid gland resulting in an adenomatous or multinodular goitre— adenomatous and colloid nodules are scattered throughout the gland. The gland may become acutely painful if haemorrhage occurs into a cyst. As the thyroid gland enlarges it may cause pressure symptoms such as dysphagia and stridor, especially if it is retrosternal.
- Thyroid malignancy.
- Thyroiditis.

Comparison of thyrotoxicosis and hypothyroidism		
Feature	Thyrotoxicosis	Hypothyroidism
Symptoms	intolerance of heat, weight loss, increased appetite, tremor, palpitations, diarrhoea, sweating, anxiety, oligomenorrhoea	intolerance of cold, weight gain, lethargy, constipation, dry skin and hair, hoarse voice
Signs	goitre, tachycardia, atrial fibrillation, warm and moist palms, tremor, Graves' disease (exophthalmos, lid lag, ophthalmoplegia)	pallor, slow pulse, thickened dry skin and hair, periorbital puffiness, loss of outer one-third of eyebrows, peripheral oedema, slow recovery phase to ankle jerk
Causes	Graves' disease, secondary thyrotoxicosis in adenomatous goitre	thyroiditis, post-thyroid surgery
Diagnosis	$\uparrow$ T$_4$ or T$_3$, $\downarrow$ TSH; Graves' disease—presence of LATS	$\downarrow$ T$_4$, $\uparrow$ TSH; Hashimoto's thyroiditis— $\uparrow$ levels of antimitochondrial antibody or antithyroglobulin antibody
Management	carbimazole or propylthiouracil, propranolol for $\uparrow$ heart rate, tremor, radioiodine, subtotal thyroidectomy	thyroxine replacement

Fig. 33.1 Comparison of thyrotoxicosis and hypothyroidism.

SOLITARY THYROID NODULE

Differential diagnosis of a solitary thyroid nodule consists of:
- Thyroid cyst.
- Benign adenoma.
- Thyroid malignancy.

Diagnosis of a solitary thyroid nodule is aided by performing an ultrasound, which can differentiate cystic from solid lesions and nodules from diffuse thyroid enlargement. A technetium-99m pertechnetate isotope scan can be used to differentiate hot and cold nodules. Inactive nodules (cold) corresponding to isolated nodules are indicators of a cyst or a tumour.

If there is a solitary solid lesion it is investigated by fine-needle aspiration cytology (FNAC). If abnormal cells are obtained then the lesion must be removed to make a precise histological diagnosis in case it is a thyroid cancer. It can be difficult to differentiate benign from well-differentiated cancers by FNAC alone.

THYROIDITIS

Autoimmune Hashimoto's thyroiditis
The patient presents with a diffuse tender goitre.

Diagnosis is made by detecting the presence of thyroid antibodies against thyroglobulin and mitochondria.

The patient is initially euthyroid and then becomes hypothyroid as the gland becomes atrophic and fibrotic. Treatment is by thyroxine replacement therapy.

Riedel's thyroiditis
This very rare condition results in a hard irregular swelling of the thyroid gland because of progressive fibrosis and may produce compression symptoms. Patients are usually euthyroid.

THYROID CARCINOMAS

Thyroid carcinomas are more common in females than males and can occur in young adults. They occur as well-differentiated adenocarcinomas of papillary, follicular or medullary type. These have a relatively good prognosis. Anaplastic carcinomas occur in the elderly and have a very poor prognosis (Fig. 33.2).

Other tumours of the thyroid, include:
- Medullary carcinoma—very rare tumour of the parafollicular or C cells of the thyroid that may arise within the syndrome of multiple endocrine neoplasia.
- Lymphoma of the thyroid—rare, but may be associated with Hashimoto's disease and is responsive to radiotherapy.

Features of main types of thyroid cancers			
Feature	Papillary	Follicular	Anaplastic
Proportion of cases (%)	60	25	10
Age	children, young adults	middle age	elderly females
Location	often multifocal	rarely multifocal	whole gland
Growth rate	slow	slow	rapid
Spread	lymphatic	blood	local infiltration causing pressure symptoms
Management	total thyroidectomy plus lymph node dissection; TSH suppression by thyroxine	thyroid lobectomy, radioactive iodine	usually inoperable; radiotherapy, chemotherapy
Prognosis	good	depends upon extent of vascular invasion	very poor

Fig. 33.2 Features of main types of thyroid cancers.

THYROID OPERATIONS

Fig. 33.3 shows a diagram of the anatomical relationships of the thyroid gland.

Indications for a thyroid operation
The common reasons for surgical intervention include:
- Subtotal thyroidectomy for control of Graves' disease.
- Relief of pressure symptoms from an enlarged multinodular goitre.
- Lobectomy or total thyroidectomy for malignant tumour.

Preoperatively the patient should be rendered euthyroid (if for Graves' disease), by prescribing carbimazole and propranolol to control symptoms.

If the patient is thyrotoxic Lugol's iodine may be prescribed for 10 days to decrease the vascularity of the gland.

Before operation the vocal cords should be inspected by direct laryngoscopy to ensure that they are functioning satisfactorily.

Operative procedure
A collar incision is made, skin flaps are elevated, and strap muscles separated to expose the thyroid gland. The middle thyroid vein is ligated and divided, the superior thyroid vessels are ligated, the thyroid lobes

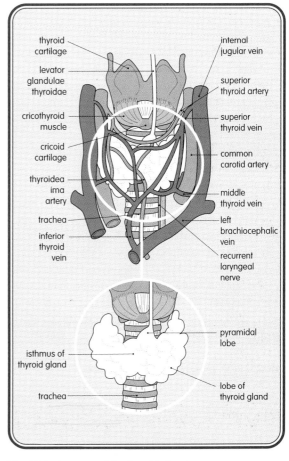

Fig. 33.3 Anatomy of the thyroid gland.

are mobilized and the recurrent laryngeal nerves and parathyroid glands are identified and preserved.

Complications of thyroid operations

These are:

1 • Immediate haematoma—may occur in the first few hours after operation. It can cause laryngeal oedema, stridor, and dyspnoea. The wound should be opened immediately, and the patient returned to theatre to control any haemorrhage.

2 • Recurrent laryngeal nerve injury—manifests as a hoarse voice or a bovine cough if one nerve is damaged. If there is bilateral damage the patient is unable to speak and any exertion causes airway obstruction. Neurapraxia usually recovers, but if there is unilateral and permanent nerve damage the cord can be injected with polytetrafluoroethylene. If both nerves are damaged an emergency tracheostomy is required.

3 • Superior laryngeal nerve (external branch) injury—produces voice changes such as loss of pitch, but it usually recovers.

4 • Hypoparathyroidism—this may be temporary or permanent. Signs of hypocalcaemia will be paraesthesia, carpopedal spasm, or Chvostek's sign of facial spasm. Immediate treatment is with calcium gluconate intravenously, followed by oral calcium and vitamin D if the response is insufficient.

5 • Hypothyroidism—if too much thyroid gland is removed then hypothyroidism develops, but if too much remains there is risk of recurrent symptoms of goitre or thyrotoxicosis.

6 • Thyroid crisis—rarely seen if the patient is euthyroid preoperatively. It may, however, be precipitated by other illnesses such as pneumonia if the patient is thyrotoxic. Symptoms are pyrexia, agitation, confusion, and tachycardia, and medication is given to control the symptoms.

PARATHYROID DISORDERS

There are four parathyroid glands:

- The superior glands arise from the fourth branchial pouch.
- The inferior glands arise from the third branchial pouch.

The parathyroid glands secrete parathyroid hormone, which:

- Stimulates osteoclastic activity in bones, which releases calcium into the circulation.
- Enhances renal tubular absorption of calcium and inhibits reabsorption of phosphate.
- Facilitates absorption of calcium from the small intestine.

HYPERPARATHYROIDISM

Background

Hyperparathyroidism can be separated into three types as outlined below.

Primary hyperparathyroidism

Primary hyperparathyroidism is due to a parathyroid adenoma or rarely a carcinoma, or due to hyperplasia of the parathyroid glands. Excess production of parathyroid hormone results in:

- Increased serum calcium and alkaline phosphatase concentration.
- Decreased serum phosphate concentration.

Secondary hyperparathyroidism

Secondary hyperparathyroidism is due to hyperplasia of the glands secondary to chronic renal failure. Renal patients have a low serum calcium due to failure of vitamin D production, which is required to absorb calcium from the gut. The resultant serum calcium may be normal or low.

Tertiary hyperparathyroidism

After renal transplantation most cases of parathyroid hyperplasia regress, but occasionally the parathyroids become autonomous and do not respond to a rising serum calcium concentration.

Clinical presentation

Clinical features of hyperparathyroidism are:

- Renal calculi..
- Bone pain—due to decalcification.
- Pathological fractures—if there is generalized cystic change of bones (i.e. osteitis fibrosa cystica).
- Muscular weakness, anorexia, intestinal atony—because of depressed nerve conduction.

- Polyuria, dehydration.
- Peptic ulceration, acute and chronic pancreatitis.
- Psychiatric disorders.

Management

A diagnosis of hyperparathyroidism is made by measuring the fasting serum calcium concentration on several occasions. It should be corrected for plasma albumin concentration. The differential diagnosis of hypercalcaemia is shown in Fig. 33.4.

Differential diagnosis of hypercalcaemia

hyperparathyroidism
ectopic parathyroid hormone secretion
  (e.g. by small cell lung tumour)
metastatic bone disease
sarcoidosis
multiple myeloma
hypervitaminosis D

Fig. 33.4 Differential diagnosis of hypercalcaemia.

Symptoms of hypercalcaemia are:
- **Bones.**
- **Stones**
- **Abdominal groans**
- **Psychic moans**

Parathyroid hormone concentration is measured by immunoassay techniques. High-resolution ultrasound or CT or MRI can be used to image the parathyroids. A thallium/technetium subtraction scan can also be used.

Parathyroid adenomas and carcinomas are treated by surgical excision.

Hyperplasia of all four glands can be treated by excision of three of the four glands. Localization of the gland at operation may be aided by an infusion of methylene blue immediately preoperatively.

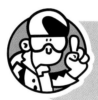

Suspect hypercalcaemia in confused, vomiting, patients who have malignant disease.

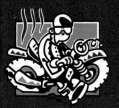

34. Neck Swellings

The anatomy of the lymphatic drainage of the neck and triangles of the neck is shown in Fig. 34.1.

CERVICAL LYMPHADENOPATHY

Background

Enlarged cervical glands may be due to a number of different pathologies:

- Primary—disorders of lymph nodes such as lymphoma. Characteristically these glands are 'rubbery', matted and large (i.e. >1–2 cm diameter).
- Secondary—to infection, which may be local or systemic (e.g.due to Epstein–Barr virus, human immunodeficiency virus). These glands are smaller, softer, and regular. The other common cause of cervical lymphadenopathy is metastatic nodes from malignant disease. Characteristically the glands are hard, irregular, and may be fixed.

Management

Any patient who has enlarged cervical nodes should have a full examination to look for other areas of lymphadenopathy or hepatosplenomegaly. Those areas that drain to the cervical nodes should be examined (including indirect laryngoscopy) for a primary lesion.

A full blood count will give information about any abnormalities of the white blood cells. Fine-needle aspiration cytology from the node will produce epithelial cells if it is a metastatic node. If the node is reactive or there is a primary lymph node problem lymphocytes will be non-diagnostic and an excision biopsy is required if a lymphoma is suspected.

If a metastatic node is identified the primary lesion may be in the:

- Larynx.
- Pharynx.
- Floor of the mouth.
- Postnasal space.

Fig. 34.1 Lymphatic drainage of head and neck.

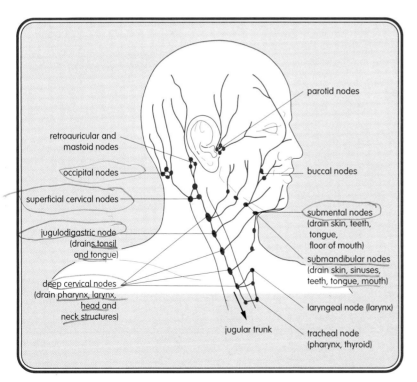

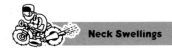
Treatment may include radical resection of the primary tumour and block resection of the lymph nodes.

If there are hard irregular metastatic nodes look for a primary lesion before excision.

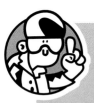

Troisier's sign is an enlarged left supraclavicular node —look for intra-abdominal pathology (due to drainage from the thoracic duct into the left subclavian vein).

OTHER CERVICAL SWELLINGS

Branchial cyst
Background
A branchial cyst arises from a congenital abnormality. In the embryo the second branchial arch grows down over the third and fourth arches to form the cervical sinus. The sinus usually disappears or may form a branchial cyst. Fig. 34.2 compares the branchial cyst with the thyroglossal cyst discussed in Chapter 33, p. 173.

Clinical presentation
A branchial cyst is often not apparent until adult life when an infection may precipitate problems. It is a soft swelling arising near the upper, anterior border of the sternocleidomastoid muscle.

Management
Aspiration of a branchial cyst shows fluid containing cholesterol crystals. The cyst can be excised to prevent further infection.

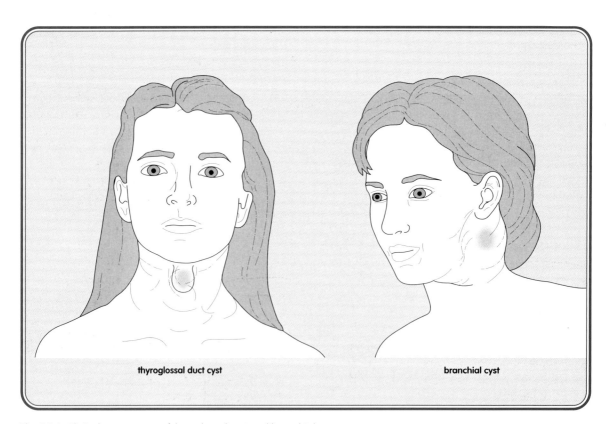

thyroglossal duct cyst

branchial cyst

Fig. 34.2 Clinical appearance of thyroglossal cyst and branchial cyst.

Branchial sinus

Failure of obliteration of the cervical sinus causes a discharging sinus anterior to the lower third of the sternocleidomastoid muscle.

Management

If the branchial sinus is excised, the track should be followed up to the side wall of the pharynx to the tonsillar fossa.

Carotid body tumour

This is a slow growing tumour arising in the carotid body at the bifurcation of the common carotid artery. The mass transmits the carotid pulsation and may be highly vascular so it demonstrates pulsation. It may be locally invasive and metastasize.

SALIVARY GLAND DISORDERS

The salivary glands commonly involved in pathological processes are the parotid and submandibular glands; the sublingual glands are rarely affected. The roles of saliva include:

- Facilitation of swallowing.
- Cleansing of mouth, gums, and teeth.
- Starch digestion (contain the enzyme ptyalin).

Salivary calculi
Background

Salivary calculi are common in the submandibular gland. The calculi develop on a nidus of debris with subsequent deposition of mucus, calcium, and magnesium phosphate.

Clinical presentation

The classic symptom of salivary calculi is a painful swelling of the gland before and during eating.

Management

On examination the gland is swollen and tender. Inspection may reveal that the duct orifice is red with a purulent discharge. Palpation of the duct may reveal the calculus, which may be visible on a radiograph of the floor of the mouth.

The calculus is removed by opening the duct or complete excision of the gland.

Acute suppurative parotitis
Background

Acute suppurative parotitis can occur in postoperative or debilitated patients who have poor oral hygiene and mouth breathing. There is usually an ascending infection caused by a staphylococcal infection.

Clinical presentation

Clinically acute suppurative parotitis is characterized by a tender inflamed swelling of the parotid.

Management

Acute suppurative parotitis is treated with antibiotics. Very rarely an abscess forms and requires drainage.

Acute parotitis may also be related to the viral infection causing mumps. In this case the swellings are usually bilateral.

Chronic parotitis

This is associated with recurrent episodes of pain and swelling of the parotid glands associated with dilatation of the duct system (i.e. sialectasia).

Sialography demonstrates the changes in the duct system.

Sjögren's syndrome
Background

Sjögren's syndrome is an autoimmune condition associated with dry eyes, xerostomia (i.e. lack of saliva), parotid swelling, and rheumatoid arthritis. It may be associated with other autoimmune conditions and it usually occurs in postmenopausal women.

Mikulicz's disease is symmetrical enlargement of the salivary and lacrimal glands caused by a benign inflammatory infiltrate and is characteristic of Sjogren's syndrome.

Management

Treatment of Sjögren's syndrome is symptomatic (i.e. artificial tears and good oral hygiene).

SALIVARY GLAND TUMOURS

There are three types of salivary gland tumour:

- Pleomorphic adenoma.
- Adenolymphoma.
- Carcinoma.

Approximately 90% of the tumours arise in the parotid gland and most of these are pleomorphic adenomas. Most patients are under 50 years of age at presentation and the majority of tumours are benign.

Pleomorphic adenoma
Background
This is usually a slow-growing smooth mass in the lower pole of the parotid gland. The tumour is lobulated with a false capsule and protrusions that go beyond the capsule. It is composed of a variety of epithelial cells with myxoid, mucoid, and chondroid elements. The mass usually arises in the superficial part of the gland.

Management
The treatment of a pleomorphic adenoma is a superficial parotidectomy. The 'tumour' should not be shelled out because some of the protrusions may be left behind and predispose to recurrence. The superficial part of the gland is removed after identification and preservation of the facial nerve.

Adenolymphoma
Background
This accounts for 10% of salivary gland tumours. It occurs in men over 50 years of age, and is occasionally bilateral. The tumours are soft and cystic.

Management
Treatment of adenolymphoma is by surgical excision and the prognosis is excellent.

Carcinoma
Background
Salivary gland carcinoma occurs in middle-aged and elderly people.

Clinical presentation
The tumours are hard, irregular, craggy lumps, and the sign of malignancy is facial nerve involvement. It may spread to the local lymph nodes, and may ulcerate. The tumours are usually squamous cell carcinomas.

Management
Treatment of salivary gland carcinoma is by radical parotidectomy (when the facial nerve may have to be sacrificed), lymph node dissection, and radiotherapy.

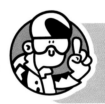

Any swelling in the parotid should be treated as a possible parotid tumour.

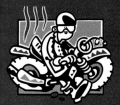

35. Breast Disorders

Breast problems account for many specialist referrals. Over 90% of them are benign, but the woman's overwhelming concern is about the possibility of breast cancer.

BREAST DEVELOPMENT

The breast develops from a breast bud, which starts to grow at puberty. It is a skin appendage consisting of fat and a major duct system leading to terminal ductolobular units. Oestrogen causes the ducts to sprout and branch at puberty, but progesterone is responsible for lobular development. The breasts increase in size because of fat deposition and connective tissue growth.

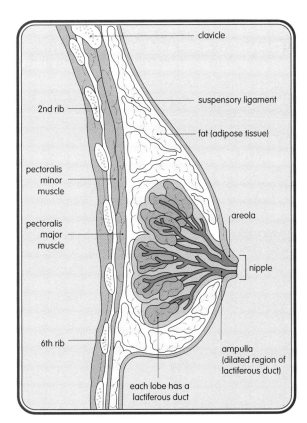

Fig. 35.1 Structure of the mature female breast.

During pregnancy there is a marked increase in the luteal and placental sex steroids, and together with human placental lactogen and chorionic gonadotrophin these lead to an increase in lobuloalveolar growth in preparation for breastfeeding. Postpartum the oestrogen levels fall and prolactin and oxytocin stimulate milk production.

The breast arises in the skin and subcutaneous tissues of the chest wall between the second and sixth ribs from the lateral border of the sternum to the mid-axillary line (Fig. 35.1).

The blood supply to the breasts is from the perforating branches of the internal thoracic, intercostal, lateral thoracic, subscapular, and thoracoacromial vessels. The lymphatic drainage follows the blood vessels to the axillary glands, supraclavicular glands, and the internal mammary glands.

Abnormalities of breast development

These include:
- Amastia—absence of the breast.
- Hypoplasia—underdevelopment of the breast.
- Virginal hypertrophy—excessive growth of the breast at puberty.
- Accessory nipples—these are very common, and are found anywhere on the milk line, which extends from the axilla to the groin.
- Accessory breast tissue—this usually occurs in the axilla, and becomes more prominent during pregnancy.
- Poland's syndrome—this is hypoplasia of the breast and chest wall (i.e. absence of the pectoralis major muscle) and the main problem is cosmetic.

BENIGN BREAST DISORDERS

Mastalgia
Background
Mastalgia (i.e. breast pain) is experienced by most women at some time in their reproductive years, but in most cases it is well tolerated. If the discomfort is cyclical (i.e. worse premenstrually) it is due to cyclical hormonal effects on the breast tissue.

Management

Cyclical discomfort is more likely than other types of mastalgia to respond to treatment such as evening primrose oil. Other simple measures include a reduction in caffeine intake. If evening primrose oil is not effective other medications that can be used are danazol and bromocriptine.

If the pain is non-cyclical and localized it may be musculoskeletal or due to costochondritis—Tietze's syndrome.

Breast infections

There are two important types of breast infection:

- Postpartum or puerperal abscess—this is associated with breastfeeding, and is usually caused by staphylococcal infection. Initially it is treated by antibiotics, but if it develops into an abscess it can be drained by percutaneous aspiration under ultrasound guidance. Occasionally it requires incision and drainage if it reaches the surface.
- Periductal mastitis—this problem usually occurs in smokers. These women experience episodes of periductal sepsis. The usual bacteria involved include anaerobes, so metronidazole is an appropriate antibiotic. The infection may resolve with antibiotics or develop into an abscess, which requires aspiration or incision, or it may discharge spontaneously to produce a fistula, which discharges intermittently at the areolar margin (Fig. 35.2).

Women who have recurrent episodes of infection need to have a total duct excision and fistulectomy for recurrent discharge.

Nipple discharge

If the discharge is green, brown, black, or cream and occurs from multiple ducts then it is due to duct ectasia (dilatation of the ducts).

Management is reassurance or total duct excision if the discharge is copious.

A blood-stained discharge from a single duct may be due to an intraduct papilloma, duct ectasia, or ductal carcinoma *in situ*. This requires exploration of the duct either by single duct excision (microdochectomy) or total duct excision.

Nipple and areola change

The areola is prone to skin changes such as eczema, which responds to 1% hydrocortisone.

The nipple may develop an erosive condition associated with underlying malignant change (i.e. Paget's disease). The nipple change is due to malignant cells spreading up the ducts. Women may present with bleeding and discharge from an ulcerated nipple, but in the early stages the areola is normal. Subsequently the nipple is destroyed and the condition spreads to the areola.

BENIGN BREAST LUMPS

The breast tissue undergoes considerable change during puberty, pregnancy, and after the age of 35 years when involution starts to occur. There are also cyclical changes due to fluctuating levels in oestrogens and progesterone. Some of the benign breast lumps that occur are just manifestations of these changes (i.e. aberrations of normal development and involution). Fig. 35.3 shows the age distribution of different types of breast lump.

Fibroadenoma

Fibroadenoma arises from the lobules and is seen predominantly in women in the 15–25-year age group during breast development. It may, however, be diagnosed at a later age when involutional changes occur.

The lump is smooth, well defined, and mobile. It is also known as a ' breast mouse ' because of its mobility.

Diagnosis is made by:

- Clinical examination.
- Characteristic ultrasound appearance.
- Benign cells on fine-needle aspiration and cytology (FNAC).

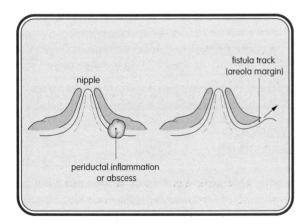

Fig. 35.2 Structure of a mammillary fistula.

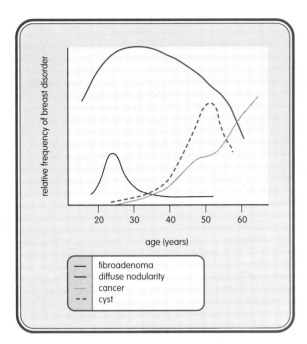

Fig. 35.3 Age distribution of different breast lumps.

Macroscopically a fibroadenoma is a well-defined encapsulated structure made up of a combination of epithelial and stromal elements.

Phyllodes tumour

This has a similar clinical appearance to that of a fibroadenoma, but develops in older women, and tends to be larger (i.e. 3–4 cm in diameter). It has malignant potential, and may develop into a sarcoma.

Breast cysts

Breast cysts are usually found in women over 35 years of age (i.e. when involutional changes occur). Microcysts form as the stroma involutes, and some of these may coalesce to form macrocysts, which may produce a palpable lump. Cysts may be single or multiple and are a feature of fibrocystic change (i.e. painful tender premenstrual nodularity).

Clinically, these cysts may seem to appear suddenly, are tender, and may resolve spontaneously. On examination there may be a well-defined smooth mass that is not mobile.

Cysts can be seen on mammograms as well-defined smooth lesions, and on ultrasound they have a characteristic appearance.

Diagnosis and treatment of a breast cyst is aspiration to extinction.

Galactocele

This is relatively uncommon, but is a cystic lump found after breastfeeding and therefore contains milky fluid.

Fat necrosis

Fat necrosis is a common sequel to trauma associated with haematoma formation. Clinically it produces a hard, irregular lump, and therefore simulates a carcinoma, but is not as common.

BREAST CANCER

Breast cancer is the commonest malignant disease of women in the UK. There are approximately 30 000 new cases of breast cancer diagnosed each year, and approximately 10 000 deaths per year. In the UK 1 in 11 women will be affected at some time in their life. The risk increases with age, and becomes more common after 50 years of age. It is more common in developed countries.

Only 1% of cases occur in men. Many of these men have female relatives affected by breast cancer, and there is often a genetic link.

Risk factors

Risk factors linked to breast cancer include:
- Genetic factors—the genes of BRCA1 and BRCA2 —account for 5% of cases, and are also linked with ovarian cancer.
- First degree premenopausal relative who has breast cancer.
- Early menarche.
- Late menopause.
- Nulliparity or late pregnancy.
- Prolonged use of hormone replacement therapy for more than 10 years.
- Benign breast pathology (i.e. atypical ductal hyperplasia and lobular carcinoma *in situ*).

Breast screening programme

In the UK all women aged between 50 and 64 years are invited for screening mammography every 3 years to detect breast cancer at an asymptomatic stage. The aim is to reduce the mortality rate from breast cancer by 30% by the year 2000.

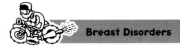

There has recently been a reduction in the mortality rate from breast cancer, but this is probably related to the increased use of adjuvant treatments.

Diagnosis of breast cancer

Important aspects in the diagnosis of breast cancer are:

- Clinical features—the obvious features are skin tethering, skin dimple, ulceration, recent nipple inversion, deep fixation, peau d'orange, and inflammatory changes. Most breast cancers do not present with advanced clinical signs and may just be a hard irregular mass or an asymmetric change in the breast.
- Imaging—mammographic features of malignancy include spiculated lesions, new mass lesions, and microcalcifications. Mammograms are not so useful in premenopausal women because of their dense glandular breast tissue. Ultrasound is useful for diagnosing benign breast lumps, cysts, and breast cancer, particularly for locating asymptomatic impalpable lesions seen on screening mammograms.
- Cytopathology—FNAC from a cancer will produce malignant cells, and core biopsies will give precise pathology.

Frozen section at operation should not be carried out because a diagnosis should be made preoperatively so that women can receive appropriate counselling.

Pathology

Aspects of the pathology of breast cancer to consider are:

- Ductal carcinoma *in situ* (DCIS; i.e. preinvasive stage of breast cancer that has not invaded the basement membrane)—after 10–15 years 50% of cases develop into invasive cancer.
- Invasive ductal carcinoma—this is the commonest type. Pathologists grade the tumours 1–3 depending upon the degree of pathological differentiation.
- Invasive lobular carcinoma—may not be visible on mammograms, and 20% of cases are bilateral. It characteristically infiltrates tissues in a diffuse manner.
- Special pathological types—these are well differentiated and should have a good prognosis (e.g. tubular, colloid, medullary, and papillary carcinomas).
- Sarcoma—very rare malignant tumour of spindle cells that may arise from a phyllodes tumour.
- Paget's disease of the nipple—usually associated with underlying neoplasm.

10% of breast cancers are not seen on mammograms.

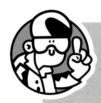

Diagnosis of breast cancer is based on triple assessment:
- **Clinical**
- **Imaging**
- **Cytology**

Treatment of breast cancer

Fig. 35.4 outlines the staging of breast cancer and 5-year survival rates. All women should have a preoperative diagnosis so that they can be given appropriate information and counselling. Many women can be given a choice of treatment. Being involved in the decision-making process can have a positive psychological effect. Some women need to be advised about treatment:

- Women are advised to have a mastectomy if there is multifocal disease, widespread DCIS, a central tumour, a large mass in relationship to the breast size (i.e. >3–4 cm in diameter).
- Women who have a locally advanced tumour or inflammatory cancer may have neoadjuvant chemotherapy in an attempt to downstage the disease before operation.
- Elderly patients who are unfit for operation may be treated with hormonal therapy (e.g. tamoxifen).
- Some women can have a choice between wide local excision, followed by radiotherapy or a mastectomy. There is no difference in the long-term survival, but there is an increased risk of local recurrence after wide local excision.
- Mastectomy may be combined with a breast reconstruction (either immediately or at a later stage) using tissue expanders or myocutaneous flaps.

A	Staging of breast cancer		
Stage	Tumour diameter	Lymph nodes	5-year survival (%)
I	<2 cm	no palpable nodes	80–90
IIA	<2 cm	palpable nodes	60–70
IIB	2–5 cm	+/– nodes	
III	>5 cm	+/– nodes	30–40
IV	advanced local disease or metastases	palpable fixed nodes	

Fig. 35.4 **(A)** Staging of breast cancer. **(B)** TNM (tumour, nodes, metastases) classification of breast cancer.

B	TNM classification of breast cancer
Classification	Criteria
Tis	ductal carcinoma *in situ*, Paget's disease of the breast
T1	tumour diameter <2 cm
T2	tumour diameter >2 cm
T3	tumour diameter >5 cm
T4	any size tumour with skin changes, fixation
N0	no regional nodal metastases
N1	metastases to ipsilateral nodes
N2	metastases to fixed nodes
N3	metastases to internal mammary nodes
M0	no distant metastases
M1	distant metastases

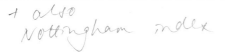

+ also Nottingham index

Prognostic factors for breast cancer are:
- **Tumour size**
- **Grade of tumour**
- **Nodal status**

Adjuvant treatment after surgery

It is now recognized that breast cancer is a systemic disease, and after operation some form of adjuvant systemic treatment should be given because it has been shown to improve the duration of disease-free survival. The type depends upon the age of the patient and the prognosis. The basic treatment regimens for different age groups are as follows:
- Premenopausal—chemotherapy +/– ovarian ablation +/– tamoxifen.
- Perimenopausal—chemotherapy or hormonal therapy.
- Postmenopausal—hormonal therapy (e.g. tamoxifen or anastrozole).

Tamoxifen blocks the oestrogen receptors on breast cancer cells. The common side effects are hot flushes and vaginal discharge, but it is usually well tolerated.

If a woman has had a mastectomy she does not require radiotherapy unless there is a high chance of local recurrence. Significant factors are tumour larger than 4 cm in diameter, vascular invasion, and more than four positive lymph nodes. In this situation the chest wall and supraclavicular nodes are irradiated.

- A radical mastectomy (Halsted's operation) with excision of pectoral muscles is only used for locally advanced disease.

Axillary surgery

The extent of operation is controversial, but lymph node status is an important prognostic indicator. Operations range from axillary node sampling to axillary node clearance.

Metastatic disease

Breast cancer cells spread by:

- Lymphatics to the drainage nodes in the axilla, internal mammary chain, and supraclavicular fossa.
- Bloodstream to the lungs, liver, bones, adrenals, and brain.
- Transcoelomic spread to produce peritoneal and pleural seedlings.
- Local spread to the chest wall, axilla, and brachial plexus.

Metastatic disease is treated symptomatically, for example:

- Radiotherapy for painful bone metastases.
- Hormone or chemotherapy for visceral metastases.
- Pleural aspiration of an effusion.
- Dexamethasone and radiotherapy for cerebral metastases.

Bone metastases may be associated with a long period of stable disease, but visceral metastases usually have a very poor prognosis.

GYNAECOMASTIA AND MALE BREAST CANCER

Gynaecomastia is the development of breast tissue in men. Aetiological factors include:

- Puberty—occurs in 30–60% of boys, but 80% regress spontaneously.
- Kleinfelter's syndrome (XXY)—lack of development of genitalia.
- Chronic liver disease.
- Hormone-secreting tumours—adrenal or testicular malignancy.
- Drugs—anabolic steroids, cimetidine, digoxin, spironolactone, oestrogens, cannabis.

The diagnosis is made by examination and exclusion of a serious underlying cause such as an adrenal tumour. Occasionally an operation is required for cosmetic reasons.

The differential diagnosis of gynaecomastia is breast cancer, but this is usually a hard craggy mass. Diagnosis is made in the same way as for women. Treatment is a mastectomy.

DDx breast lump.

1 Breast ca
2 Fibroadenoma
3 Cyst
4 Breast abscess
5. Cystosarcoma Phyllodes
6. Galactocele
7. Duct ectasia
8. Duct papilloma

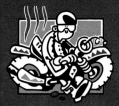

36. Vascular Disorders

Vascular problems include conditions of the veins, arteries, and lymphatics. The problems can be acute or chronic.

CHRONIC LIMB ISCHAEMIA

Background

This usually affects the lower limb, rather than the upper limb, but many patients have a history of other ischaemic problems such as angina, myocardial infarction, or cerebrovascular event. Predisposing factors for all of these conditions are:

- Atherosclerosis.
- Diabetes mellitus.
- Hyperlipidaemia.
- Family history.
- Smoking.
- Buerger's disease. = *Inflamm. arts, vs*

+ as. c thrombosis in middle +jcal arts.

Stages of ischaemia are: *found only in ♂ smokers*

- Intermittent claudication—cramp-like pain in the legs exacerbated by exercise and relieved by rest. Pain develops distal to the obstruction so blockage of the femoropopliteal segment causes calf pain, but blockage of the aorta causes buttock pain and impotence (Leriche's syndrome).
- Rest pain—implies that the ischaemia is critical and the viability of the leg is threatened. The pain is severe and requires opioid analgesia.
- Gangrene—in dry gangrene ischaemia results in death of the tissue. The tissue is black and there is a clear line of demarcation, which may separate. Wet gangrene is brown, moist, and ulcerated. The tissue is infected with pathogenic bacteria so the infection may spread proximally and can cause systemic toxicity.

Management

After the history and full examination of the cardiovascular system, blood tests are taken to:

3 cardinal features critical ischaemia =
1. Ulceration
2. gangrene
3. Pain at rest.

 # (N) = 1. Impending gangrene: ≤ 0.3

- Look for anaemia, polycythaemia, and hyperlipidaemia.
- Measure blood glucose concentration.
- Assess renal function.

The vasculature is assessed by Doppler ultrasound, ankle/brachial pressure measurement, and arteriograms (Fig. 36.1).

The treatment of chronic limb ischaemia depends upon the severity of the condition:

- Intermittent claudication—patients are advised to stop smoking, encouraged to exercise to produce an efficient oxygen extraction from the limited blood supply, and prescribed aspirin 75 mg/day. On this regimen 60% of patients will improve or remain stable.
- Critical ischaemia—any exacerbating factors such as infection are treated. Arteriography is performed to define the extent and position of the occlusion. A single short segment, less than 5 cm long can be treated by balloon angioplasty and with a success rate of more than 85% and a 1-year patency of more than 70%. Alternatively an expandable metal stent can be used.

If the arteriograms show multisegment disease then revascularization is performed by reconstructive surgery. Aortoiliac disease is treated by using a synthetic bifurcated graft from the aorta to both femoral vessels distal to the obstruction (Fig. 36.2).

If the patient is unfit for a major abdominal operation then a graft can be passed from the axillary artery to the femoral vessels under local anaesthetic.

Femoropopliteal disease is bypassed using the patient's own long saphenous vein (reversed) or a synthetic graft.

For grafts to be successful there should be good inflow and good distal run-off. There is a risk of occlusion in the immediate and later postoperative periods. Aspirin is prescribed to decrease the risk of thrombosis, but if the patient continues to smoke there is a high risk of graft failure.

Signs
Absent pulses
1. cold white legs
2. atrophic skin
3. punched out ulcers
4. postural colour change

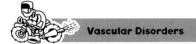
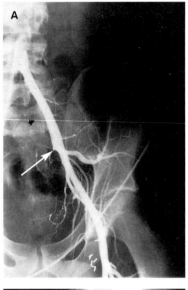

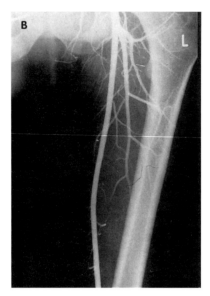

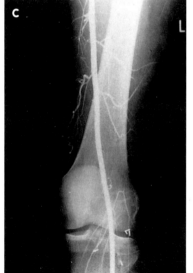

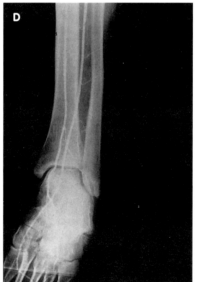

Fig. 36.1 Arteriogram showing occlusion of the internal iliac artery (arrow) and good flow to the leg. **(A)** View of external iliac artery. **(B)** View of superficial femoral artery. **(C)** Popliteal artery. **(D)** Distal vessels to lower leg and foot.

ACUTE LIMB ISCHAEMIA

Background

Acute limb ischaemia can occur in the upper or lower limbs and is usually due to an embolus or thrombosis or vascular injury.

Clinical presentation

The history is of sudden onset of a painful cold limb. The presence of paraesthesia indicates severe ischaemia and once mottling occurs this heralds gangrene. Muscle rigidity implies that the damage is irreversible.

Clinical features of acute ischaemia—6 Ps:
- Pulselessness
- Pain
- Pallor
- Perishing cold
- Paraesthesia
- Paralysis

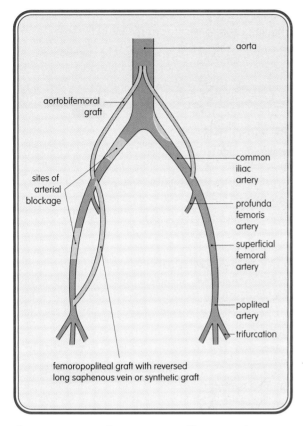

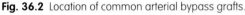

Fig. 36.2 Location of common arterial bypass grafts.

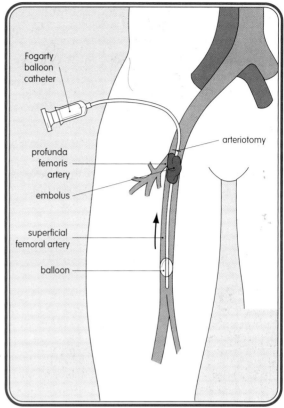

Fig. 36.3 Use of Fogarty balloon catheter to extract an embolus from the superficial femoral artery.

If there is no history or signs of previous vascular insufficiency then an embolus is suspected. The common causes are an embolus:

- From a mural thrombus in the right atrium, associated with atrial fibrillation.
- A thrombus may develop over an area of myocardial infarction.

Rarer sites of an embolus are from the valves, a ventricular aneurysm, an atrial myxoma, or an atheromatous plaque.

If there is a past history of ischaemia then the problem is probably acute on chronic (i.e. a thrombosis).

Vascular injury may also occur after trauma or after an intervention such as an arteriogram.

Management

Once the diagnosis is suspected the patient is anticoagulated with intravenous heparin to prevent further thrombosis. If the clinical picture suggests an embolus then an urgent embolectomy can be performed under local anaesthetic. A Fogarty balloon catheter is used to extract the embolus (Fig. 36.3). Postoperatively the patient is anticoagulated to prevent recurrence.

If the history suggests an underlying vascular problem and there are signs of chronic ischaemia an arteriogram is required to define the problem. Thrombolytic therapy such as streptokinase, urokinase, or tissue plasminogen activator may be infused locally to lyse the thrombus. It may take 12–72 hours to be effective so cannot be used if the viability of the limb is threatened.

It may be necessary to carry out a reconstructive operation to revascularize the limb.

COMPARTMENT SYNDROME

Background

A complication of acute ischaemia is compartment syndrome. Ischaemia and reperfusion of the muscles causes them to swell within their rigid osseofascial compartment. Further increase in pressure exceeds capillary perfusion pressure so the blood supply is impaired causing further ischaemia and swelling.

Clinical presentation

Clinically the patient has severe pain, especially on moving the muscles of the affected compartment. An urgent fasciotomy is required to open the compartment and allow the muscles to expand. If the muscle is damaged it releases myoglobin, which can cause renal damage, and ischaemia causes lactic acid production and metabolic acidosis.

ANEURYSM

This is an abnormal dilatation of a vessel, which can occur at several different sites in the body (e.g. abdominal or thoracic aorta, iliac, femoral, popliteal, or cerebral arteries). The different types of aneuryms are illlustrated in Fig. 36.4. The common causes are:
- Congenital—berry aneurysm in the circle of Willis.
- Atherosclerotic—commonest.
- Traumatic—after interventional radiology or trauma.
- Inflammatory—mycotic or syphilitic.

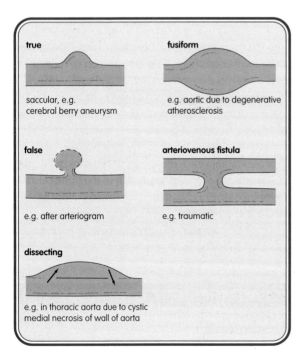

true

saccular, e.g. cerebral berry aneurysm

fusiform

e.g. aortic due to degenerative atherosclerosis

false

e.g. after arteriogram

arteriovenous fistula

e.g. traumatic

dissecting

e.g. in thoracic aorta due to cystic medial necrosis of wall of aorta

Fig. 36.4 Types of aneurysm.

All aneurysms can rupture, thrombose, be a source of embolus, cause pressure symptoms, or become infected.

ABDOMINAL AORTIC ANEURYSM

Background

Abdominal aortic aneurysm is the commonest type of aneurysm and the incidence is increasing. Most are associated with smoking, atherosclerosis, and hypertension. They usually extend from just below the renal arteries to the bifurcation of the aorta, but some patients also have aneurysms of the iliac vessels.

Clinical presentation

An abdominal aortic aneurysm may present in a variety of ways as follows:
- It may be asymptomatic—being detected during a routine physical examination or abdominal ultrasound examination or abdominal radiography because 50% are calcified.
- As an abdominal pulsation.
- With recent onset of severe back pain—may be due to an enlarging aneurysm eroding the vertebrae.
- With back or flank pain (may be similar to ureteric colic) and episodes of hypotension—due to a leaking retroperitoneal aneurysm.
- With circulatory collapse and severe abdominal pain—due to an intraperitoneal rupture.
- With congestive cardiac failure, abdominal bruit, lower limb ischaemia, and oedema—due to erosion into the inferior vena cava.

Management.

In the non-acute situation a diagnosis of abdominal aortic aneurysm is made by an ultrasound scan, but a computed tomography (CT) scan gives better definition of renal artery involvement, and acutely it may confirm a retroperitoneal haematoma, implying a leak. Aneurysms over 5 cm in diameter have a high risk of rupture.

If surgical resection is contemplated patients should have a detailed cardiorespiratory assessment. If an aneurysm is repaired electively it is replaced with a synthetic graft and 95% of patients survive. If the aneurysm ruptures many patients do not reach hospital and 50% do not survive the operation, so the overall mortality rate is 85%.

If patients survive the operation there may be complications related to underlying cardiac, respiratory, or renal disease and problems related to clotting abnormalities.

Repair of the aneurysm may cause acute lower limb ischaemia due to embolus or thrombosis, colonic ischaemia, or spinal cord ischaemia. *prevent by clamping overflow vessel*

Late complications are graft infection, aortoenteric fistula, and development of a false aneurysm at the site of the anastomoses.

THORACOABDOMINAL ANEURYSM

Background
A thoracoabdominal aneurysm can involve the ascending and descending thoracic aorta, and the abdominal aorta.

Clinical presentation
A thoracoabdominal aneurysm may be asymptomatic, but severe chest, back or abdominal pain indicates expansion and impending rupture.

Management
A chest radiograph shows a widened mediastinum or calcification of the aortic wall. A CT scan defines the extent of the aneurysm:
- Type A dissection of ascending aorta—needs aortic arch replacement—very poor outcome.
- Type B dissection of descending aorta—treat with conservative control of blood pressure.

DIABETIC FOOT PROBLEMS

Background
Diabetics have an increased risk of ulceration and infection of the feet because of their predisposition to:
- Atherosclerosis affecting the large vessels.
- Microangiopathy (i.e. thickening of the basement membrane of the small arterioles and capillaries).
- Neuropathy of the sensory, motor, and autonomic systems.
- Increased risk of infection because a glucose-rich environment favours bacterial growth.

Management of diabetic's foot
Treatment of diabetic's foot involves:
- Clinical assessment.
- Radiography to look for osteomyelitis and soft tissue damage.
- Antibiotics to treat bacterial infection after swabs for culture.
- Assessment of arterial circulation—using Doppler or arteriogram.
- Good diabetic control.

Neuropathic ulcers will heal after treatment of infection and debridement of any necrotic tissue.

Ischaemic ulcers will only heal if the arterial supply improves.

Fig. 36.5 gives a comparison of the features of ischaemic and neuropathic ulcers.

Comparison of features of ischaemic and neuropathic ulcers		
Feature	Ischaemic ulcers	Neuropathic ulcers
Sensation	painful	sensory impairment
Pulses	absent or decreased	present
Ulceration	on toes and pressure areas	plantar ulceration—deep, painless
Temperature of foot	cold	warm due to autonomic neuropathy
Other features	variable sensory changes, intermittent claudication	trophic skin lesions, Charcot's joints

Fig. 36.5 Comparison of features of ischaemic and neuropathic ulcers.

The best management of the diabetic foot is patient education and prevention.

AMPUTATION

Despite aggressive surgical intervention some patients who have atherosclerotic or diabetic problems either present too late or the reconstructve procedures fail and their tissues bcome ischaemic and die. This causes severe pain and there is often superimposed infection so amputation is the only treatment left to relieve their symptoms and prevent further complications.

The type of amputation depends upon the level of an adequate blood supply to allow the wound to heal.

Types of amputation include:

- Above knee.
- Below knee.
- Syme's amputation through the talotibial joint.
- Forefoot amputation.
- Digital amputation.

Following amputation there should be an active rehabilitation programme of physiotherapy and occupational therapy to encourage the patient to have a prosthesis and return to the community. Many patients, however, experience severe phantom limb pain and their underlying disease progresses so that they require a further operation and many die within a few years.

CAROTID ARTERY DISEASE

Background

Many patients who have peripheral vascular disease also have atherosclerosis affecting the carotid artery. They usually have hypertension and are smokers. Men are affected more often than women and patients are usually over 65 years of age at presentation.

Clinical presentation

Patients may present with:

- A transient ischaemic attack (TIA, i.e. transient loss of sensory or motor function) or amaurosis fugax (temporary blindness), which last for less than 24 hours.
- A cerebrovascular event ('stroke').

Management

Clinical examination may demonstrate a bruit over the carotid vessels, but this is not always the case. Duplex scanning of the carotid arteries can detect stenosis and digital subtraction arteriography will demonstrate the anatomy. If a patient has had a 'stroke' a CT scan can show whether it is due to infarction or haemorrhage.

If there is evidence of carotid artery stenosis general measures are to stop smoking and control hypertension, diabetes mellitus, and hyperlipidaemia.

Antiplatelet drugs such as aspirin decrease the risk of TIA and 'stroke'.

An operation is performed if the patient is symptomatic and the stenosis is over 70%. A carotid endarterectomy is performed to remove the atheromatous plaque. There is a small risk of cerebral damage, but usually the operation is successful.

CORONARY ARTERY DISEASE

Background

This is due to atherosclerosis of the coronary arteries. Risk factors are:

- Smoking.
- Hypertension.
- Hyperlipidaemia.
- Obesity.
- Diabetes mellitus.

Clinical presentation

Coronary artery disease may present with angina or a myocardial infarction.

Management

Coronary angiography is performed to assess the problem. If there is triple vessel disease or stenosis of the left anterior descending coronary artery (LAD) coronary artery bypass grafts are required. The internal thoracic artery is anastomosed to the LAD and long saphenous vein can be used for other grafts. This operation has a 1–4% hospital mortality rate, but only 50% of vein grafts are patent at 10 years and 10% of patients will have a second operation within 10 years.

THROMBOANGIITIS OBLITERANS

Background
Thromboangiitis obliterans (Buerger's disease) is a condition that usually affects young men who are smokers. It is characterized by segmental thrombotic occlusions of small- and medium-sized vessels in the upper and lower limbs. There is an associated inflammatory infiltrate, which affects the arteries, veins, and occasionally the nerves.

Clinical presentation
Patients present with symptoms of peripheral vascular disease, which is progressive unless they stop smoking.

RAYNAUD'S DISEASE

Background
This occurs in young women who have no underlying vascular diseases.

Clinical presentation
Patients who have Raynaud's disease have an exaggerated response to the cold. The fingers become white because of ischaemia, blue because of cyanosis, and then red from hypaeremia. This is often associated with pain and paraesthesia.

Management
Treatment is:
- Avoidance of the cold.
- Stop smoking.
- Reassurance.

Nifedipine may be useful.

Late-onset Raynaud's phenomenon is associated with an underlying cause.

RAYNAUD'S PHENOMENON

Background
This occurs in older people than Raynaud's disease and is associated with:

- Autoimmune conditions such as polyarteritis nodosa and rheumatoid disease.
- Malignancy.
- Myeloproliferative disorders.
- Vibration tools.
- Scleroderma.

Unilateral Raynaud's phenomenon
This may be associated with subclavian embolic disease or thoracic outlet compression syndrome and there may be neurological signs. This problem is due to a cervical rib compressing the axillary vascular bundle and lower brachial plexus.

Clinical presentation
The neurological symptoms of unilateral Raynaud's phenomenon are worse when the arm is abducted and externally rotated.

Management
Treatment of unilateral Raynaud's phenomenon is excision of the cervical rib and resection of the subclavian aneurysm.

VARICOSE VEINS

Background
Varicose veins are tortuous, dilated, superficial veins that have incompetent valves. The long and short saphenous veins in the legs are usually involved. Varicose veins are common, but most are relatively asymptomatic.

Some people have a congenital malformation of the veins (Klippel–Trénaunay syndrome), which comprises varicose veins, limb hypertrophy, and a port wine stain.

Most cases of varicose veins are idiopathic or familial, but some are secondary to a previous deep vein thrombosis. In women the veins get worse with each pregnancy because of impaired venous return and progesterone-induced dilatation of the veins.

Normally blood drains from the superficial to the deep veins by the action of the contracting muscles. At several points there are perforating veins with valves, which regulate one-way flow. If the valves become incompetent, especially at the junction of long saphenous vein and femoral vein, the blood refluxes back into the superficial veins and they become varicose.

In the postphlebitic limb the deep veins are thrombosed so all the blood returns via the superficial veins and if there is recanalization the valves are damaged.

Clinical presentation

Many patients are asymptomatic, but others are aware of aching discomfort and swelling of the legs, and are concerned about the appearance. Complications of the veins are:

- Varicose eczema.
- Ulceration secondary to poor capillary circulation.
- Oedema of the skin and therefore poor nutrition to the skin.

At the point where the perforators and the superficial veins meet there are often blowouts (i.e. bulbous dilatation of the vein). In the groin this is called a saphena varix. These dilatations may bleed if traumatized. Thrombophlebitis can occur.

Management

Clinical examination will define the extent of the problem, the veins affected, and the levels of the incompetent valves. If there is a history of thrombosis a venogram must be performed to ensure that the deep veins are patent. A duplex scan is also used to demonstrate the level of incompetent valves.

Many patients are advised about support hosiery. Indications for operation are complications such as bleeding and ulceration.

The saphenofemoral junction is the main point of incompetence so the long saphenous vein and the associated tributaries are disconnected from the femoral vein (high tie).The thigh segment of the long saphenous vein may be stripped, other perforators are ligated, and other segments of the vein can be avulsed. Postoperatively the patients wear support hosiery for several weeks and exercise.

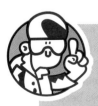

Deep vein thrombosis and superficial thrombophlebitis may precede the clinical presentation of a cancer, especially pancreatic cancer.

Injection sclerotherapy is only suitable for small veins. The veins are injected with a sclerosant, which causes a chemical thrombophlebitis to occlude the vein.

SUPERFICIAL THROMBOPHLEBITIS

This is local inflammation of a superficial vein and may develop secondary to prolonged cannulation or infusion of an irritant substance or it may occur in varicose veins.

Thrombophlebitis migrans comprises recurrent episodes of superficial thrombophlebitis and may precede clinical manifestations of malignancy or be associated with connective tissue disease.

SUBCLAVIAN OR AXILLARY VEIN THROMBOSIS

Background

Prolonged arm exercises may precipitate subclavian or axillary vein thrombosis as a result of repetitive venous occlusion, or the thrombosis may develop spontaneously or secondary to cannulation.

Clinical presentation

The arm is painful and swollen and there are prominent superficial collateral veins.

Management

Treatment is systemic anticoagulation.

LYMPHATIC DISORDERS

Lymphoedema
Background
A complex system of lymphatic channels drains the subcutaneous tissues. The channels from the legs pass via the lymph node groups to the cisterna chyli and the thoracic duct to return to the venous system. If this transport system fails the protein-rich fluid accumulates in the subcutaneous tissues:

- Primary lymphoedema is a congenital abnormality and may present at birth, in adolescence, or in middle age, depending upon the degree of the abnormality of the lymphatic system.

- Secondary lymphoedema occurs after interruption or blockage of the lymphatic channels by surgical excision, infection, tumour infiltration, or radiotherapy. Worldwide filarial worm is the commonest cause.

Clinical presentation

Whether the lymphoedema is primary or secondary, the limb is swollen and heavy. Initially the oedema is pitting, but then it becomes fibrosed. The situation is worsened by recurrent episodes of infection (i.e. lymphangitis).

Management

Treatment comprises advice about exercise, massage, compression hosiery, and external pneumatic compression to control the swelling.

A rare event is the development of a malignant tumour within the lymphoedema after more than 10 years. This is a lymphangiosarcoma that presents with reddish blue discoloration or nodules and has a very poor prognosis.

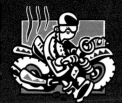

37. Urological Disorders

URINARY TRACT INFECTION

Urinary tract infection (UTI) is seen in many medical disciplines and in all age groups:

- In children it may be due to a congenital abnormality or vesicoureteric reflux and needs to be investigated to prevent long-term damage.
- In young adults women are affected more than men because of a short urethra.
- At all ages strictures and stones predispose to infection.
- In elderly men infection is secondary to outflow obstruction.

Diagnosis is confirmed by mid-stream urine (MSU) and culturing more than 10^5 organisms/mL. Usual organisms are:

- *Eschericha coli*—80% of cases of cystitis and pyelonephritis.
- *Enterobacter* and *Klebsiella* spp.—hospital-acquired infections.
- *Pseudomonas* and *Candida* spp.—immunosuppressed patients or after antibiotics.
- *Proteus* spp.—often associated with urinary calculi.

Acute cystitis
Patients who have acute cystitis have symptoms of:
- Frequency.
- Urgency.
- Dysuria.
- Suprapubic pain.
- Malaise.
- Haematuria.

Treatment is oral antibiotics.

Acute pyelonephritis
Clinical presentation
The symptoms of acute pyelonephritis are:
- Pyrexia.
- Loin pain.
- Dysuria.
- Rigors.
- Malaise.

Management
On examination the patient is pyrexial and has loin tenderness.

Diagnosis is by MSU and blood cultures. An ultrasound and intravenous urogram (IVU) are used to look for any underlying cause.

Treatment of acute pyelonephritis is with intravenous antibiotics because of the risk of septicaemia. If the infection is inadequately treated it may form a renal abscess, which may develop into a perinephric abscess.

Chronic pyelonephritis
Recurrent infections of the kidney cause chronic inflammation and glomerular fibrosis and may present as hypertension and renal impairment.

Xanthogranulomatous pyelonephritis
This is an extreme form of chronic pyelonephritis. There is an excessive inflammatory response with lipid-laden macrophages, and multiple parenchymal abscesses. Renal function is poor and treatment is often a nephrectomy.

Acute bacterial prostatitis
The symptoms of acute bacterial prostatitis are those of a UTI with low back pain and perineal discomfort. On examination the prostate is tender.

Treatment is with intravenous antibiotics and then a prolonged course of oral antibiotics to prevent development of an abscess.

Chronic bacterial prostatitis
Chronic bacterial prostatitis may follow acute infection. The symptoms are painful micturition with perineal pain. An MSU should be taken after prostatic massage. Treatment is long term oral antibiotics.

RENAL TRACT CALCULI

Background
Factors predisposing to renal tract calculi are:
- Inadequate drainage—such as pelviureteric junction (PUJ) obstruction, bladder diverticulum, abnormal anatomy of renal tract.
- Excess of normal constituents—increased calcium (as a result of hyperparathyroidism, sarcoidosis, immobilization), uric acid (after chemotherapy), hyperoxaluria, cystinuria, hyperuricosuria.
- Abnormal constituents—UTI, foreign body, hyperkeratosis of epithelium (e.g. vitamin A deficiency), renal tubular acidosis, medullary sponge kidney.

Common reasons for calculi are:
- **Idiopathic hypercalciuria**
- **UTI**

90% of renal calculi are calcified.

Clinical presentation
Ureteric calculi may be asymptomatic, or cause haematuria and ureteric colic, which is a severe colicky pain radiating from the loin to the groin and penis or labium. The haematuria may be macroscopic or microscopic.

Management
A diagnosis of ureteric calculus is based upon the typical history, detection of haematuria, and an IVU defines the level of obstruction. Blood tests and a 24-hour urine collection are performed to look for underlying biochemical abnormalities.

Initial treatment is with analgesia, and non-steroidal anti-inflammatory drugs such as diclofenac sodium have been found to be effective.

Most calculi less than 6 mm in diameter in the lower urinary tract pass spontaneously. If they do not and

there are any signs of infection urgent intervention is required to extract the calculus. Calculi tend to lodge at the PUJ, pelvic brim, and vesicoureteric junction, and may cause hydronephrosis and hydroureter with a risk of pyonephrosis.

Treatment of calculi
Renal stones can be fragmented by extracorporeal shock wave lithotripsy (ESWL) so that they will pass down the ureter. Occasionally the stone is too large and does not respond to ESWL so it is removed by percutaneous nephrolithotomy. Under general anaesthetic a nephroscope is inserted to fragment and remove the stone. The kidney is drained by a nephrostomy tube and a nephrostogram is performed to ensure that the ureter is clear of calculi before it is removed.

Open operation may be necessary to remove a staghorn calculus, which is usually seen in women who have had recurrent UTIs. The calculus consists of calcium, ammonium, and magnesium phosphate. *Proteus* spp. splits urea to form ammonium salts. The problem may be asymptomatic until renal damage occurs. If the stone is large it may have to be removed by pyelolithotomy or nephrolithotomy, or nephrectomy if renal function is severely impaired.

Ureteric calculi can be removed using the ureteroscope. The calculus can be pushed back to the renal pelvis and then undergo ESWL or be disintegrated by a lithotrite. The stone may be retrieved by a dormia basket. Occasionally a ureterolithotomy (open surgery) is necessary.

Bladder calculi
Bladder calculi form in a neuropathic or obstructed bladder, and diverticula. Schistosomiasis and UTI predispose to their formation. They may cause acute retention. Treatment is stone retrieval by cystoscopy and cystolithotomy.

A filling defect on an IVU may be due to:
- **Radiolucent stone**
- **Ureteric malignancy**

RENAL CARCINOMA

Background
This is an adenocarcinoma arising from the proximal convoluted tubules. Macroscopically it is yellow because of its lipid content. It spreads locally through the capsule and along the vein, metastasizes to lymph nodes, and bloodborne metastases are distributed to the lungs and bones.

Clinical presentation
This includes:
- Haematuria.
- Loin pain.
- Abdominal mass.

Systemic effects include anaemia, pyrexia of unknown origin, and metabolic disturbances of calcium, ectopic adrenocorticotrophic hormone or antidiuretic hormone secretion, polycythaemia, and coagulopathy.

Renal carcinoma can cause a left varicocele if the renal vein is obstructed.

Renal carcinoma may also be an asymptomatic discovery on an ultrasound scan or present with metastases.

Management
If a diagnosis of renal carcinoma is suspected the kidney is imaged by CT scan and this will stage the tumour. The function of the opposite kidney is assessed. A chest radiograph may show cannon ball metastases.

The staging of renal carcinoma is:
- I—tumour confined to the kidney.
- II—tumour extends through the capsule.
- III—tumour extends to the renal vein, nodes, or fascia.
- IV—distant metastases or local invasion.

Treatment is by radical nephrectomy. It may be possible to resect solitary lung metastases. Hormone and chemotherapy are not effective, but immunotherapy is under investigation. Overall survival is 40% at 5 years.

NEPHROBLASTOMA (WILMS' TUMOUR)

This is a malignant tumour occurring in children under 5 years of age. It may present as an abdominal mass or pain.

Diagnosis is made by ultrasound or CT scan.

Treatment is a combination of surgery, chemotherapy, and radiotherapy to produce a cure rate of 80%.

TUMOURS OF THE RENAL PELVIS AND URETER

Transitional cell carcinomas of the renal pelvis and ureters are rare. They can present with painless haematuria, clot colic, loin pain, or be associated with transitional cell carcinoma of the bladder.

Diagnosis is made from urine cytology, IVU, CT scan, and ureteroscopy.

Treatment is nephroureterectomy.

BLADDER CANCER

Background
The incidence of bladder cancer is increasing. It is predominantly a transitional cell carcinoma. Aetiological factors include smoking, and association with the dye and rubber industries (e.g. naphthylamine).

Squamous cell carcinoma is rare except where schistosomiasis is endemic.

Adenocarcinoma is very rare and is associated with a persistent urachal remnant. Fig. 37.1 shows the staging and prognosis of bladder cancer.

Management
Bladder cancer usually presents with painless haematuria (95% of cases). Carcinoma *in situ* may produce symptoms similar to those of a UTI, but no haematuria. Investigations include:
- MSU and urine for cytology.
- IVU.
- Cystourethroscopy.

CT scan and transvesical ultrasound can be used to assess the depth of the tumour.

Superficial tumours—T0 and T1
These are diagnosed by multiple biopsies to assess the depth. The tumour is resected via a cystoscope (i.e. transurethral resection of tumour—TURT) and patients are reviewed regularly to look for further tumour. Recurrence occurs in 50%. Risk factors for local recurrence are smoking and large and multiple tumours.

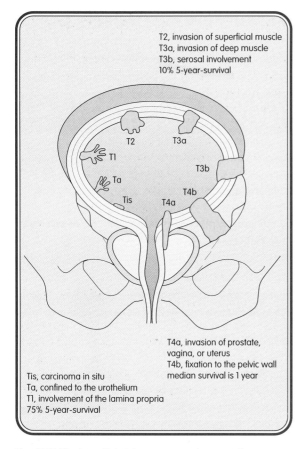

T2, invasion of superficial muscle
T3a, invasion of deep muscle
T3b, serosal involvement
10% 5-year-survival

T2
T3a
T1
T3b
Ta
T4b
Tis
T4a

T4a, invasion of prostate, vagina, or uterus
T4b, fixation to the pelvic wall median survival is 1 year

Tis, carcinoma in situ
Ta, confined to the urothelium
T1, involvement of the lamina propria
75% 5-year-survival

Fig. 37.1 Staging of bladder cancer and prognosis.

If there is evidence of carcinoma *in situ* or there is a high-grade superficial tumour or frequent recurrence then treatment with intravesical chemotherapy may be used.

Invasive tumours—T2 and T3

More radical treatment is required for these tumours, such as radical radiotherapy or a radical cystectomy with formation of an ileal conduit. Radiotherapy may result in the side effects of cystitis and proctitis, and make later operation more difficult.

Locally advanced and metastatic tumours may benefit from chemotherapy.

PROSTATIC CANCER

Because the population is ageing prostatic cancer is becoming more common. It is an adenocarcinoma that arises in the glandular epithelium at the periphery of the gland.

Histologically prostatic cancer is classified using the Gleason grading system for the degree of differentiation. It spreads locally via the lymphatics and bloodstream.

The symptoms of prostatic cancer are those of bladder outflow obstruction or of metastatic bone disease.

Management

Clinical examination reveals a hard, irregularly enlarged prostate with obliteration of the median sulcus. Blood tests are used to check the renal function and measure prostatic-specific antigen (PSA).

Transrectal ultrasound can be used to image the prostate and to guide a trucut biopsy. Abdominal ultrasound will reveal signs of bladder outflow obstruction such as hydronephrosis and residual urine volume. A bone scan can be carried out to look for bone metastases, which are usually sclerotic deposits on plain radiographs.

Treatment is as follows:
- Bladder outflow obstruction—transurethral resection.
- Localized tumours (T1 or T2)—radiotherapy or radical prostatectomy.
- T3 or T4 tumours—radiotherapy, which may produce complications of prostatitis or cystitis.
- Metastatic disease—hormonal manipulation because the tumour is androgen dependent. Methods of treatment include bilateral subcapsular orchidectomy, luteinizing hormone releasing hormone agonists, or antiandrogens such as cyproterone or flutamide.

Fig. 37.2 shows the staging of prostatic cancer and prognosis.

Most bladder cancers are transitional cell carcinomas except where schistosomiasis is endemic.

Prostatic cancer tends to produce sclerotic metastases.

TESTICULAR CANCER

Primary testicular cancer develops in young men. Risk factors include cryptorchidism or undescended testis, even after fixation.

Teratoma and seminoma account for 90% of testicular tumours:

- Teratomas occur in 20–30 year olds.
- Seminomas occur in 30–50 year olds.

Both types metastasize to the para-aortic nodes because the testes originate from that area.

Testicular lymphoma may occur in older men and treatment is as for lymphoma in other sites.

Management

Testicular cancer usually presents as a painless irregular and hard swelling of the testis.

The diagnosis is made by ultrasound of the testis and measurement of the tumour markers α-fetoprotein and β-human chorionic gonadotrophin. A chest radiograph is taken to look for metastatic disease and abdominal CT is used to stage the disease and look for para-aortic nodes.

Once the diagnosis is made an orchidectomy is performed using an inguinal approach so that the cord and vessels are clamped before handling the testis to prevent dissemination. Further treatment depends upon the stage.

With improvement in diagnosis, staging, and treatment overall cure rates can be as high as 90%, and if the patient is node negative it can be 100%. Fig. 37.3 shows the staging and management of testicular tumours.

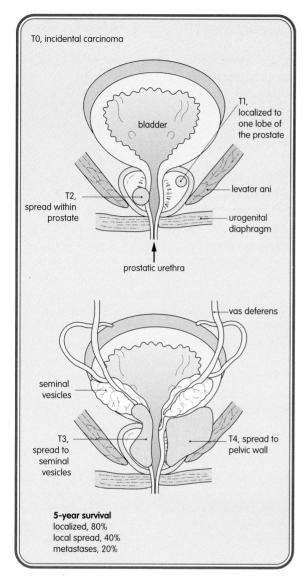

Fig. 37.2 Staging of prostatic cancer and prognosis.

Staging of testicular tumours and management			
Stage	Definition	Management of teratoma	Management of seminoma
I	confined to testis	orchidectomy and observe or RPLND	orchidectomy and radiotherapy to para-aortic nodes
II	retroperitoneal nodes	chemotherapy and RPLND to residuum	radiotherapy to nodes
	bulky disease		radiotherapy plus chemotherapy
III	nodal disease above diaphragm	chemotherapy	radiotherapy to nodes plus chemotherapy
IV	visceral metastases	chemotherapy	chemotherapy

Fig. 37.3 Staging of testicular tumours and management. (RPLND, retroperitoneal lymph node dissection.)

PENILE CANCER

This is rare in the UK, but is most likely to occur in uncircumcised elderly men. It is a squamous cell carcinoma, that spreads locally to the inguinal nodes. It presents as a painful ulcerating lesion on the penis or enlarged nodes.

The treatment depends upon the size of the lesion at presentation:

- Surgical treatment can range from a circumcision to partial or complete amputation of the penis.
- Radiotherapy may be used for small lesions on the glans.
- A block dissection of the nodes is the best treatment for involved nodes.

LOWER URINARY TRACT OBSTRUCTION

Fig. 37.4 shows the causes of lower urinary tract obstruction.

Obstructive symptoms are:
- Weak stream.
- Hesitancy.
- Intermittent stream.
- Dribbling.
- Straining.

Irritative symptoms are:
- Frequency.
- Urgency.
- Nocturia.
- Urge incontinence.

Benign prostatic hypertrophy

Benign prostatic hypertrophy (BPH) develops in the central part of the gland, initially in the periurethral glands. Changes occur with advancing years, but the precise reason for these changes is unknown. Patients have a combination of symptoms of obstruction and irritation.

Intermittent stream, terminal dribbling, and incomplete emptying occur when the detrusor is unable to maintain sufficient pressure to overcome the obstruction. Chronic retention may develop with a large residual volume and overflow incontinence.

Acute urinary obstruction may be precipitated by a UTI or drugs such as α-adrenergic, anticholinergic, and psychotropic drugs.

Fig. 37.5 shows the effects of bladder outflow obstruction.

Fig. 37.4 Causes of lower urinary tract obstruction.

Causes of lower urinary tract obstruction	
Disorder	Causes
meatal stenosis	congenital in newborn or infant males; balanitis in adults
urethral stenosis	trauma or inflammation in females; instrumentation or venereal disease in males
posterior urethral valves	congenital mucosal folds in young males
spasm of urethral sphincter	spinal cord injury, multiple sclerosis
benign prostatic hypertrophy	elderly males
prostatic cancer	elderly males
bladder neck contracture	usually secondary to trauma or operation
cystocele	women who have had a vaginal delivery or a pelvic operation
detrusor inhibition	anticholinergic agents such as phenothiazines, antianxiolytic drugs
systemic neurological conditions	Guillain–Barré syndrome, diabetes mellitus, uraemia, and chronic alcoholism can affect the autonomic nervous system

Management

Examination of a patient who has lower urinary tract obstruction may demonstrate a palpable bladder, and an enlarged smooth prostate.

Investigations include MSU for infection and haematuria and tests of renal function. An ultrasound of the pelvis will reveal a residual volume after micturition and any pressure effects on the kidneys. A urine flow measurement gives an objective assessment of symptoms. A cystoscopy is carried out to detect any associated bladder lesions.

The most effective treatment is transurethral resection of prostate (TURP). Occasionally a very large gland requires an open retropubic prostatectomy.

Complications of TURP include haemorrhage, clot retention, and TURP syndrome, which is due to systemic absorption of the bladder irrigation fluid. It causes a hyponatraemic, hypochloraemic metabolic acidosis, hypo- or hypertension, tachycardia, and confusion. Late complications of TURP are impotence, incontinence, and urethral stricture.

Alternative treatments for BPH include adrenergic blockers, which act on the prostatic smooth muscle and capsule. Drugs that convert testosterone to dihydrotestosterone (e.g. finasteride) may decrease the size of the gland.

Other new techniques include transurethral stents, balloon dilatation, and microwave or ultrasound hyperthermia.

Some patients have a combination of neurological and obstructive symptoms so are unsuitable for operation and catheterization is more appropriate.

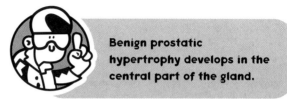

Benign prostatic hypertrophy develops in the central part of the gland.

UPPER URINARY TRACT OBSTRUCTION

If urine flow is obstructed it causes renal impairment. The ipsilateral blood flow decreases, but the contralateral flow increases to compensate. If the obstruction is not relieved renal damage occurs due to pressure and ischaemia.

Acute renal failure needs to be managed by dialysis and percutaneous nephrostomy before definitive treatment of the obstruction.

Fig. 37.6 shows the causes of upper urinary tract obstruction.

RENAL TRANSPLANTATION

Patients who have chronic renal failure due to chronic pyelonephritis, diabetes mellitus, hypertension, polycystic kidneys, or connective tissue disorders are maintained on dialysis until a kidney becomes available.

The transplant can be from a cadaver or a living related donor provided there is ABO blood group compatibility and human leucocyte antigen (HLA) tissue type compatibility.

The kidney is transplanted into the pelvic area and the renal vessels are anastomosed to the iliac vessels. The ureter is implanted into the bladder.

hydroureter— leading to hydronephrosis and renal failure

diverticulum— residual urine leading to UTI and calculus formation

trabeculation— due to muscle hypertrophy

haematuria— fragile veins are damaged at the end of micturition

enlarged prostate

urethral compression— resulting in a diminished stream

Fig. 37.5 Effects of bladder outflow obstruction.

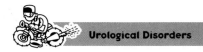

Causes of upper urinary tract obstruction		
Location	Cause	Notes
within the lumen	calculi	
	clot	
	renal papillary necrosis	due to diabetes mellitus, sickle cell anaemia or analgesic abuse
within the wall	PUJ obstruction	m>f; young adults have loin pain after a fluid load; diagnosed by IVU; treatment is pyeloplasty to resect abnormal PUJ
	ureteric tumour	presents with pain and haematuria; diagnosed by IVU and cytology
	vesicoureteric junction obstruction	congenital in boys; symptoms are pain and haematuria; treatment is ureteric reimplantation
	ureteric stricture	due to trauma, surgical manipulation, pelvic radiotherapy or chronic inflammation; treatment is resection
extraluminal	vascular abnormalities	
	neoplastic tumours in pelvis	cervical, bladder, prostate, rectal, ovarian, and uterine tumours
	retroperitoneal fibrosis	idiopathic or due to radiotherapy or malignant tumour; symptoms are ↑ BP, loin pain, and renal impairment; on IVU the ureters are pulled medially and there is hydronephrosis; treatment is stent insertion and then an operation to free the ureters from the obstruction (ureterolysis)

Fig. 37.6 Causes of upper urinary tract obstruction. (f, female; IVU, intravenous urography; m, male; PUJ, pelviureteric junction.)

Complications include rejection, acute or late, acute tubular necrosis, and infection. Following operation patients require lifelong immunosuppressive medication with azathioprine, corticosteroids, and cyclosporin.

Graft survival is 80% at 1 year and 60% at 5 years.

URINARY INCONTINENCE

Background

Incontinence is involuntary loss of urine and it may be stress induced (i.e. induced by coughing, laughing, or lifting). It usually affects multiparous women and is due to urethral incompetence.

Urge incontinence is due to unstable detrusor contractions and is associated with frequency and urgency. This may be due to a neuropathic bladder or an unstable detrusor and is exacerbated by infection, calculi, and tumours.

Constant incontinence can be due to an ectopic ureter or a ureterovaginal fistula, which can develop after a hysterectomy, birth trauma, or pelvic radiotherapy. In the elderly it may be due to immobility or impaired mental function.

Management

The patient is examined to look for a cystocele, palpable bladder, or enlarged prostate. Other tests include an MSU, IVU, and urodynamic assessment. Videocystometry will show unstable contractions and stress incontinence.

Urge incontinence is managed by:
- Treating any underlying cause.
- Prescribing drugs that relax the smooth muscle.
- An operation may be carried out to distend the bladder or increase the bladder size by augmentation with the caecum.

Stress incontinence is managed by:

- Bladder exercises.
- Drugs that increase the bladder neck closure.
- Operation to lift the bladder neck and urethral suspension.
- An artificial urinary sphincter may be necessary.

TESTICULAR PROBLEMS

Undescended testis

The testis develops on the posterior abdominal wall and descends after the processus vaginalis and gubernaculum into its position in the scrotum. Its progress may be halted or altered so that the testis remains intra-abdominal, inguinal, or high in the scrotum. It may not be palpable and ultrasound or CT scan may be needed to identify it.

If the testis fails to descend by 1 year of age it should be surgically moved (i.e. orchidopexy). If it remains in an abnormal position the seminiferous tubules are damaged and there are risks of infertility and malignant change and it is more prone to trauma.

Torsion of the testis

This is a problem of teenage boys and young adults and may be due to abnormal mesentery on the testis. The history is of an acute onset of scrotal pain, which may be associated with lower abdominal pain and vomiting. There may be a history of preceding episodes that resolved. On examination the scrotum will be red, and the testis will lie horizontally and be very tender. If diagnosis is delayed there may be inflammation and a reactionary hydrocele.

If torsion is a possibility it requires urgent exploration. If the testis is already infarcted it is removed. If it is viable after untwisting both testes are fixed. Even after 4 hours damage will have occurred to spermatogenesis, but the hormonal function may be preserved.

The differential diagnosis of torsion includes torsion of the hydatid of Morgagni, which is an embryological remnant on the testis.

Epididymitis presents a similar picture, but is unusual in adolescents.

Epididymo-orchitis

Sexually transmitted infection or UTI may precipitate epididymo-orchitis. Orchitis may be secondary to viral infection of mumps and appears 3–4 days after parotitis.

Symptoms of epididymo-orchitis are a painful testis and epididymis, with pyrexia, malaise, and features of UTI. The scrotum is red, inflamed and tender.

The organisms involved are *Chlamydia trachomatis* or *Neisseria gonorrhoeae* if due to sexually transmitted infection, but Gram-negative organisms if it is secondary to a UTI.

Epididymo-orchitis is treated with appropriate antibiotics.

SCROTAL PROBLEMS

The differential diagnoses for a scrotal mass are described in Fig. 37.7.

Hydrocele

This is a collection of fluid in the tunica vaginalis surrounding the testis. It may be congenital if seen in boys under 1 year of age and is due to persistent patency of the processus vaginalis. Most close spontaneously.

In adults it may be primary and idiopathic or develop secondary to infection, tumour, or trauma. An ultrasound will reveal any underlying pathology and the hydrocele should be treated accordingly.

Idiopathic hydrocele can be treated by excision or plication of the sac.

Epididymal cyst

Cysts commonly arise from the epididymis. They may be single or multiple thin-walled cysts felt separately from the testis. If it contains sperm it is a spermatocele. Most are asymptomatic and can be left. If multiple cysts are excised there is a risk of damaging the epididymis.

Urgent exploration is essential for suspected torsion of the testis.

Varicocele

This is an abnormal dilatation of the veins of the pampiniform plexus, which is more common on the left than right. It may be a presentation of renal carcinoma.

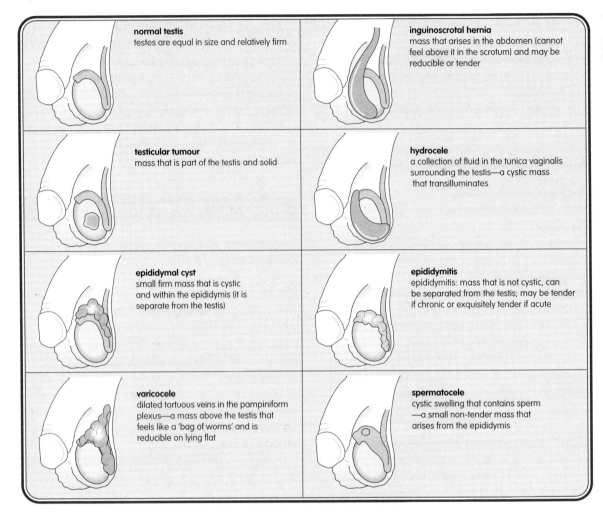

Fig. 37.7 Differential diagnosis of a scrotal mass.

Symptoms of a varicocele are a dragging sensation and heaviness in the scrotum. The veins are prominent on standing and feel like a ' bag of worms'. The main reason for seeking advice is infertility.

A varicocele can be treated by ligation of the testicular veins at the level of the deep inguinal ring.

DISORDERS OF THE PERINEUM

The disorders of the perineum are:
- Balanitis—an infection of the foreskin, which is usually due to staphylococci. It affects young boys and may cause retention because of the pain and swelling. It is treated with antibiotics.
- Phimosis—tightness of the foreskin so it will not retract. It is treated by circumcision.

- Paraphimosis—the foreskin is retracted behind the glans and cannot be reduced so forms a constriction band and the glans swells. Treatment is reduction by gentle traction and later circumcision.
- Hypospadias—a congenital condition in which the urethral opening is in an abnormal position on the ventral position of the penis or scrotum. Severe forms need surgical correction.
- Fournier's gangrene—a severe synergistic infection of the perineal tissues, which may develop secondary to perianal sepsis or periurethral sepsis. It causes gangrene of the overlying tissues, which requires radical debridement of the subcutaneous tissues.
- Scrotal cancer—rare squamous cell cancer related to exposure to soot and poor hygiene.

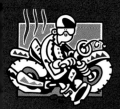

38. Skin Lesions

The different types of skin lesions to be discussed in this chapter are shown in Fig. 38.1.

BENIGN CONDITIONS

Sebaceous cyst
Background
This cyst is caused by obstruction of a sebaceous gland.

NO – Derived from hair follicle

Clinical presentation
Sebaceous cysts are common on the scalp, head, neck, and trunk. They form well-defined cystic lesions in the epidermis, which have a central punctum and contain 'cheesy material' of epidermal debris.

Management
Sebaceous cysts are treated by excision to prevent the complications of infection, ulceration, or calcification.

Lipoma
Background
A lipoma is a subcutaneous lobulated mass of fat that has a thin capsule.

Clinical presentation
Lipomas can occur intramuscularly and retroperitoneally, where they may develop into liposarcomas. The presence of multiple lipomas may be familial and this is known as Dercum's disease.

Dermoid cyst
Background
A congenital dermoid cyst forms when the embryological folds fuse (i.e. angular dermoids above the eyebrows or midline dermoids). Occasionally a midline dermoid communicates with a cyst in the anterior fossa of the skull.

Clinical presentation
The cysts consist of epidermal cells and lie deep to the skin.

An implantation dermoid is a cystic lesion that has developed following trauma (e.g. a puncture wound that implants epidermal cells into the subcutaneous tissues).

Hidradenitis suppurativa
Background
This is a condition affecting the sweat glands that results in recurrent infections and sinuses, which discharge.

Clinical presentation
Hidradenitis suppurativa occurs in the axilla, groins, and perineum.

Fig. 38.1 Types of skin lesions.

Types of skin lesions	
Type	**Examples**
benign conditions	sebaceous cyst, lipoma, dermoid cyst, hidradenitis suppurativa
benign skin tumours	papilloma, wart, pyogenic granuloma, histiocytoma (dermatofibroma), neurofibroma, keratoacanthoma, seborrhoeic keratoses, solar keratosis
vascular lesions	strawberry naevus, capillary haemangioma, cavernous haemangioma, lymphangioma, glomus body tumour
malignant skin lesions	basal cell carcinoma, squamous cell carcinoma, Kaposi's sarcoma, Bowen's disease
pigmented lesions	naevi, malignant melanoma

Management
Minor episodes resolve spontaneously, but abscesses may require incision and drainage. Chronic widespread problems are treated by excision of the affected skin, which is left open to heal by granulation tissue.

BENIGN SKIN TUMOURS

Papilloma
A papilloma is an overgrowth of skin that produces a sessile or pedunculated polyp.

Wart
Background
Warts are caused by viruses that produce papillary hyperplasia and excessive keratinization.

Clinical presentation
Warts are commonly seen on the hands and feet (e.g. verrucas). Sexually transmitted disease of the perineum is due to human papillomavirus.

Management
Wart treatments include salicylic acid, cryotherapy, podophyllin, and silver nitrate.

Pyogenic granuloma
Clinical presentation
This lesion usually develops after trauma and is an exuberant mass of granulation tissue, which bleeds easily.

Management
Pyogenic granuloma can be excised under local anaesthetic.

Histiocytoma
Background
Histiocytoma (dermatofibroma) is a very common skin nodule caused by infiltration by lipid-filled macrophages.

Clinical presentation
Clinically histiocytoma is a firm hemispherical nodule.

Management
Diagnosis and treatment of histiocytoma is by excision.

Neurofibroma
This is a small firm subcutaneous mass. It is a benign nerve sheath tumour. Multiple neurofibromas with café-au-lait spots are a feature of neurofibromatosis (von Recklinghausen's disease), which is an autosomal dominant condition.

Keratoacanthoma
Background
The history for a keratoacanthoma is that of a rapidly growing lump over a period of 6 weeks, which ulcerates and then regresses and heals over 2–3 months.

Clinical presentation
Keratoacanthoma is often found on the face and hands. An important differential diagnosis is squamous cell carcinoma.

Seborrhoeic keratoses
Background
These are very common in elderly people, especially on the trunk.

Clinical presentation
Seborrhoeic keratoses are raised and pigmented and have a waxy feel. Histologically they consist of stratified squamous epithelium.

Solar keratosis
Background
Solar keratosis is very common in elderly people and arises in areas exposed to the sun.

Clinical presentation
The lesions consist of hyperkeratosis and are premalignant.

Management
Solar keratosis should be excised and advice given about decreasing sun exposure.

VASCULAR LESIONS

Strawberry naevus
Background
Strawberry naevus (capillary cavernous haemangioma) occurs about 10 days after birth and rapidly enlarges to several centimetres in diameter.

Clinical presentation
A strawberry naevus is a vascular lesion that appears red, raised, and compressible. It regresses spontaneously over a period of several years to leave a small scar.

Capillary haemangioma
Clinical presentation
Capillary haemangioma (port wine stain) can occur at any site, but may correspond to a sensory dermatome.

Management
Attempts to remove a capillary haemangioma cause scarring so cosmetic camouflage is required.

Capillary haemangioma may be associated with a central nervous system lesion (i.e. Sturge–Weber syndrome).

Cavernous haemangioma
Background
This is a localized collection of dilated veins.

Clinical presentation
Cavernous haemangioma is a bluish–purple lesion.

Management
Cavernous haemangiomas are excised because of the risk of ulceration and bleeding.

Lymphangioma
Clinical presentation
This consists of lymphatic channels, which contain clear fluid. The largest form is a congenital cystic hygroma of the neck.

Glomus body tumour
Background
A glomus body tumour is an arteriovenous formation that is sensitive to temperature.

Clinical presentation
It is usually seen on the digits as a purplish lesion beneath the nails.

Management
Glomus body tumours are exquisitely tender and should be removed.

MALIGNANT SKIN LESIONS

Over the past 10 years there has been an increased incidence of malignant skin lesions because of increased exposure to ultraviolet radiation, but also increased public awareness for detecting early change. Predisposing factors for the development of malignant lesions are:
- Exposure to sunlight.
- Radiation exposure.
- Chemical carcinogens (e.g. arsenic, coal tar, oils).
- Inherited disorders (e.g. xeroderma pigmentosa).
- Chronic ulceration (e.g. Marjolin's ulcer).

Basal cell carcinoma (rodent ulcer)
Background
Basal cell carcinoma is a malignant tumour of the basal cells of the epidermis. It invades locally, but does not metastasize.

Clinical presentation
Basal cell carcinoma is a common lesion, especially on the forehead, nose, and face, but can occur in many different sites. The characteristic appearance is of an ulcerated lesion with a rolled, pearly margin and telangiectasia.

Management
Treatment of basal cell carcinoma is surgical excision or radiotherapy.

Squamous cell carcinoma
Clinical presentation
Squamous cell carcinoma is an ulcerated lesion with everted edges. It spreads locally, but also metastasizes to regional nodes.

Management
Diagnosis is by biopsy and treatment is surgical excision or radiotherapy.

Kaposi's sarcoma
Background
This is an angiomatous neoplasm affecting the skin.

Clinical presentation
Kaposi's sarcoma is purple and occurs on the hands and feet. It is now a common presentation of acquired immunodeficiency syndrome (AIDS).

Bowen's disease
Background
Bowen's disease is a premalignant change
(i.e. squamous carcinoma *in situ*).

Clinical presentation
Bowen's disease produces a raised red, hyperkeratotic,
well-demarcated lesion.

Management
The lesion can be treated by 5-fluorouracil or
cryotherapy, but surgical excision is preferable.

PIGMENTED LESIONS

Naevi are benign pigmented lesions that develop from
increased numbers of melanocytes. There are several
different types depending upon the position of the
melanocytes including:
- Lentigo—the melanocytes are in the basal layer of
  the epidermis. This is usually seen on the face.
- Junctional—the melanocytes are at the junction of
  the dermis and epidermis. These arise before
  puberty, and are smooth and flat.
- Intradermal—the melanocytes are in the dermis.
  This is an elevated lesion and is the commonest
  variety.
- Compound—the melanocytes are at the junction
  and in the dermis. This has a mixed appearance
  and may become malignant.
- Blue—the melanocytes are deep in the dermis.

The signs indicating malignant changes in naevi are
listed in Fig. 38.2

**Any suspicious lesion should
be excised for precise
histological diagnosis.**

Malignant melanoma
Clinical presentation
A melanoma is usually a brown–black pigmented
irregular lesion and may show evidence of bleeding or
ulceration, but can be amelanotic.

Signs of malignant change of naevus

new lesion
increased size, colour, and pigmentation
bleeding, crusting, ulceration
pain, itching
satellite lesions
lymphadenopathy

Fig. 38.2 Signs of malignant change in a naevus.

Malignant melanomas are commonly found on the
lower limbs, feet, head, and neck. The two common
types are:
- Superficial spreading malignant melanoma.
- Nodular malignant melanoma.

Initially the malignant cells spread laterally and
then they grow vertically and have the potential
to metastasize via the lymphatic system or
bloodstream to the liver, bone, brain, lungs, and
gastrointestinal tract.
  Other types of malignant melanoma are:
- Acral lentiginous melanoma, which can occur on the
  soles of the feet.
- Subungal melanoma.

Management
A melanoma is assessed by pathologic assessment
of the depth of the tumour according to Breslow's
classification or Clarke's levels.
  A poor prognosis is associated with melanomas that
are ulcerated, greater than 4 mm in depth, occur on the
trunk or in men.
  Surgical excision is the main treatment.
  Subungal melanoma is treated by excision of the digit.
  If there are involved nodes a block dissection should
be performed.
  Local recurrence or satellite nodules without distant
metastases are treated by perfusing the limb with a
chemotherapy agent (melphalan) at 42°C (i.e. isolated
hyperthermic limb perfusion).
  The role of immunotherapy such as interferon is
being investigated because melanoma is not responsive
to chemotherapy or radiotherapy.
  Fig. 38.3 shows the recommendations for surgical
excision margins and the prognosis for different stages
of melanoma.

A melanoma < 0.75 mm in depth has a very good prognosis, but if it is > 4 mm in depth it has a very poor prognosis.

 Sites of malignant melanomas that have a poor prognosis are the BANS:
- Back of the arm
- Neck
- Scalp

Recommendations for surgical excision margins and prognosis for melanoma		
Breslow thickness	Excision margin	5-year survival (%)
In situ	clear margins	100
<1 mm	1 cm	95–100
1–2 mm	1–2 cm	80–95
2.1–4 mm	2 cm	60–75
>4 mm	2–3 cm	50

Fig. 38.3 Recommendations for operative excision margins and prognosis for melanoma.

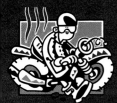

39. Soft Tissue Disorders

Ingrowing toe nail
Background
Ingrowing toe nails are common, especially in adolescents, and they usually affect the hallux of the foot.

Clinical presentation
The nail edge starts to grow into the adjacent soft tissue and there may be superimposed infection, so cellulitis and granulation tissue develop. Simple measures to improve foot hygiene include cutting the nail transversely so that the nail does not grow into the soft tissues. An operation may be needed involving:

- Wedge resection (Fig. 39.1)—removal of the edge of the nail and phenolization of the nailbed to prevent regrowth.
- Zadik's operation—excision of the whole nail and nailbed to stop regrowth.

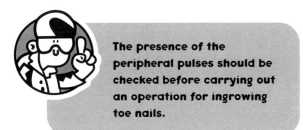

The presence of the peripheral pulses should be checked before carrying out an operation for ingrowing toe nails.

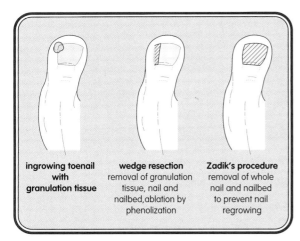

| ingrowing toenail with granulation tissue | wedge resection removal of granulation tissue, nail and nailbed, ablation by phenolization | Zadik's procedure removal of whole nail and nailbed to prevent nail regrowing |

Fig. 39.1 Operative treatment for ingrowing toenails.

Paronychia
Clinical presentation
Paronychia is an infection of the soft tissue at the edge of the nail and commonly occurs in the fingers.

Management
An abscess develops, which requires incision and drainage.

Onychogryphosis
Clinical presentation
Onychogryphosis is a deformity of the nail, especially the hallux of elderly people. The nail is very thickened and twisted.

Management
If the nail is avulsed it will regrow in the same way and the only treatment is complete removal and ablation of the nailbed—Zadik's operation.

Dupuytren's contracture
Clinical presentation
Dupuytren's contracture is thickening and contracture of the palmar or plantar aponeurosis. It causes flexion of the digits at the metacarpophalangeal and proximal interphalangeal joints. In most cases it is idiopathic, but it can be familial or associated with liver disease, epilepsy, and the use of phenytoin.

Management
Treatment is by fasciectomy to straighten the flexed fingers.

Ganglion
Clinical presentation
A ganglion is a benign myxoma of the joint capsule or tendon sheath and is commonly found on the hand or wrist, dorsum of the foot, or peroneal tendons of the ankle. It is a soft protrusion from the synovial sheath surrounding a tendon or a joint capsule. It has a synovial lining and contains synovial fluid. It can fluctuate in size so treatment may not be necessary.

Management

The ganglion can be excised, but will recur if the communication with the capsule or sheath is not identified.

PILONIDAL SINUS

Clinical presentation

A pilonidal sinus ('nest of hairs') occurs in the natal cleft of young hairy males, but it may occur between the fingers in hairdressers. It is due to hairs getting into the skin and causing an inflammatory reaction. In the natal cleft there are central pits with lateral sinuses, which discharge, or an abscess develops.

Management

Abscesses are incised and drained, but the whole sinus and its tracts should be excised to prevent recurrence.

SOFT TISSUE TUMOURS

Clinical presentation

Young people who present with a short history of an intramuscular mass should be suspected of having a malignant tumour (e.g. liposarcoma, rhabdomyosarcoma, chondrosarcoma, lymphoma).

Management

The differential diagnosis includes a lipoma or other benign tumour. Common sites for soft tissue tumours are the limbs, pelvic girdle, and retroperitoneum.

Diagnosis is made by imaging by ultrasound, magnetic resonance imaging, or computed tomography to assess the site and extent of the mass (Fig. 39.2).

An image-guided trucut biopsy can be obtained to provide a tissue diagnosis:

- If it is malignant the patient is assessed for metastatic disease.
- If a solitary sarcoma is identified and it is deemed operable (i.e. it does not invade the neurovascular bundle), it is excised radically (i.e. compartment excision or excision of the whole muscle to completely excise the tumour without breaching

its capsule). This may be preceded or followed by radiotherapy or chemotherapy to decrease its size.

The prognosis depends upon the size, grade, degree of differentiation, and excision margins of the tumour.

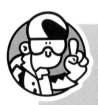

A diagnosis of sarcoma should be suspected in any patient who presents with a new intramuscular mass.

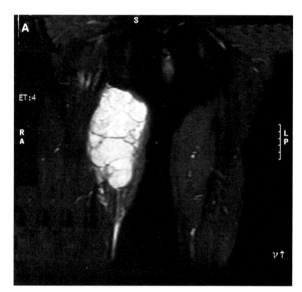

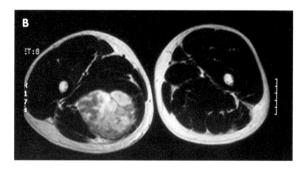

Fig. 39.2 Magnetic resonance images of thigh showing sarcoma of the thigh. **(A)** Longitudinal view. **(B)** Cross-sectional view.

40. Trauma

Trauma is the leading cause of death in the first four decades of life. Death may occur at one of three stages:

- Within minutes of the injury—if there is laceration of the brain or brainstem or spinal cord injury, or damage to the heart and major vessels.
- From a few minutes to a few hours after trauma —the 'golden hour'—with rapid assessment and appropriate management deaths can be avoided.
- Several days to weeks after injury—this is usually due to sepsis and organ failure.

The quality of the initial assessment is vital to sustaining life and the quality of life.

The primary survey and management of trauma patients are outlined Fig. 40.1.

Assessment includes a history of the mechanisms of the injury because this gives clues about the likely injuries.

Background information on the patient's general health may influence further management.

It is important to assess the vital signs rapidly, and maintain oxygenation and circulation because early death is due to uncontrollable haemorrhage and hypoxia leading to irreversible organ failure.

Fig. 40.2 shows the areas of possible injury. Once the patient is more stable a full secondary survey occurs to look for the non-life-threatening injuries.

A classification of hypovolaemic shock is given in Fig. 40.3.

O-negative blood can be used while awaiting crossmatch.

Management of trauma patients

primary survey
    A—airway maintenance and cervical spine control
    B—breathing and ventilation
    C—circulation and haemorrhage control
    D—disability and neurological status
resuscitation
secondary survey
definitive care

Fig. 40.1 Management of trauma patients.

CHEST INJURIES

Tension pneumothorax
Background
This occurs when the lung is damaged by a penetrating injury, which then acts as a one-way valve so that the air escapes from the lung into the pleural cavity (Fig. 40.4), causing collapse of the lung, mediastinal shift, decreased venous return, and decreased ventilation of the opposite lung.

Management
The diagnosis is made clinically based upon the following signs:
- Severe respiratory distress.
- Tracheal deviation.
- Unilateral absence of breath sounds.
- Cyanosis.
- Distended neck veins.
- Hypertympanic percussion note.

Treatment is immediate decompression by insertion of a chest drain.

Open pneumothorax
Background
If there is a large open defect in the chest wall there is a pneumothorax, but the air is able to escape so the pressure does not increase so rapidly.

Management
The defect in the chest wall should be sealed with dressings and a chest drain inserted.

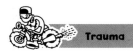

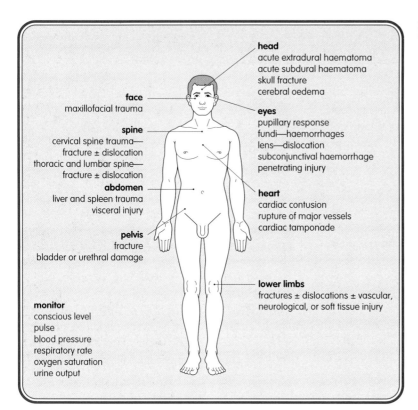

Fig. 40.2 Sites of possible traumatic injuries.

head
acute extradural haematoma
acute subdural haematoma
skull fracture
cerebral oedema

face
maxillofacial trauma

eyes
pupillary response
fundi—haemorrhages
lens—dislocation
subconjunctival haemorrhage
penetrating injury

spine
cervical spine trauma—
fracture ± dislocation
thoracic and lumbar spine—
fracture ± dislocation

abdomen
liver and spleen trauma
visceral injury

heart
cardiac contusion
rupture of major vessels
cardiac tamponade

pelvis
fracture
bladder or urethral damage

lower limbs
fractures ± dislocations ± vascular,
neurological, or soft tissue injury

monitor
conscious level
pulse
blood pressure
respiratory rate
oxygen saturation
urine output

Classification of hypovolaemic shock		
Class	Blood loss	Clinical features
I	<15%	minimal symptoms and signs
II	15–30% (800–1500mL)	pulse rate >100, ↑ respiratory rate, ↓ blood pressure and ↓ urine output
III	30–40%	tachycardia, tachypnoea, confusion, ↓ blood pressure and ↓ urine output
IV	>40%	life-threatening—skin cold and pale, tachycardia, low blood pressure, oliguria, ↓ conscious level
	50%	loss of consciousness, pulse and blood pressure

Fig. 40.3 Classification of hypovolaemic shock.

Shock is defined as acute circulatory failure with inadequate tissue perfusion causing cellular hypoxia.

Clinical presentation
There are signs of hypovolaemia and respiratory impairment. A chest radiograph will show fluid in the pleural cavity.

Management
The patient should be resuscitated and a chest drain inserted. If the blood loss is more than 200mL/h a thoracotomy is performed to control haemorrhage.

Haemothorax
Background
After blunt or penetrating injury, intrathoracic structures may be damaged resulting in a haemothorax.

Flail chest
Background
If there are multiple rib fractures the normal movement of the chest wall is disrupted (see Fig. 40.4).

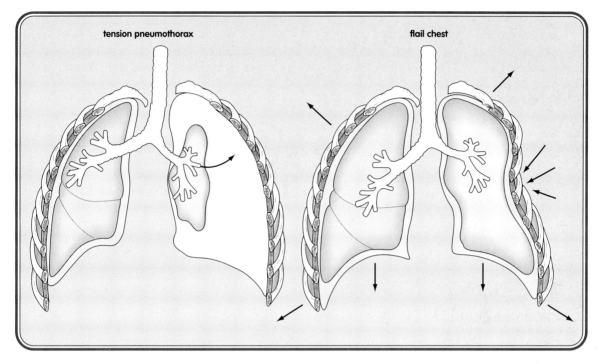

Fig. 40.4 Tension pneumothorax and flail chest. In a tension pneumothorax air escapes from the lung into the pleural cavity. A flail chest results from multiple rib fractures, which disrupt the normal movement of the chest wall.

Clinical presentation
The underlying lung is usually damaged causing hypoxia. The injured chest wall moves paradoxically (i.e. not with the rest of the chest wall), so the chest movement is decreased and further hypoxia develops.

Management
The patient may need ventilation to maintain oxygenation until the ribs stabilize.

Simple pneumothorax
Background
A fractured rib may penetrate the lung resulting in a pneumothorax and lung collapse.

Clinical presentation
The patient is breathless.

Management
A chest radiograph confirms the diagnosis and a chest drain is inserted in the fourth or fifth intercostal spaces anterior to the axillary line.

Cardiac tamponade
Background
This is usually caused by penetrating injury, but may be due to major blunt trauma.

Clinical presentation
Blood in the pericardium depresses the cardiac output and increases the venous pressure.

Management
The diagnosis is based upon the signs of a decreased blood pressure and heart sounds, but increased venous pressure.

Treatment is urgent pericardiocentesis (i.e. aspiration of the pericardial sac).

Traumatic aortic rupture
Background
Approximately 90% of these injuries are fatal at the site of the accident, but if the adventitial layer remains in tact rupture is delayed.

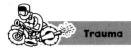

Management
Diagnosis is suspected if there is a widened mediastinum. A CT scan or aortography confirms the diagnosis and urgent surgical repair is then required.

Oesophageal rupture
Background
Oesophageal rupture is usually due to penetrating trauma.

Clinical presentation
It is suspected by the presence of surgical emphysema in the neck, a left pneumothorax, and mediastinal air on chest radiography.

Management
Treatment is urgent surgical exploration.

Diaphragmatic rupture
Background
This is more common on the left side and is caused by blunt trauma causing radial tears leading to herniation.

Clinical presentation
A diaphragmatic rupture may go unnoticed until the patient develops bowel obstruction many years later.

Pulmonary and myocardial contusion
Background
Trauma to the chest wall usually causes damage to the underlying lung, which may cause respiratory failure 24 hours after injury even if the ribs are not injured.

Clinical presentation
Myocardial contusion causes chest wall pain and abnormalities on the electrocardiogram (ECG).

Management
Myocardial contusion may predispose to important arrhythmias. Treatment is supportive.

Rib fracture
Background
Relatively minor trauma can fracture ribs in the elderly. The pain of rib fracture inhibits ventilation, so may cause hypoxia especially if the patient had underlying lung disease.

Clinical presentation
If the first and second ribs are fractured there is often marked major injury to the head, neck, spinal cord, lungs, and great vessels. In young people fractures of ribs 4–9 are most common.

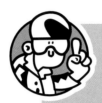

Life-threatening thoracic conditions are:
- **Tension pneumothorax**
- **Cardiac tamponade**
- **Open chest wound**
- **Massive haemothorax**
- **Flail chest**

ABDOMINAL TRAUMA

Background
Blunt or penetrating injuries or compression against the vertebral column can cause marked internal damage. A penetrating injury requires a laparotomy because of the risk of visceral injury.

Management
Patients who have a blunt injury should be carefully assessed and re-evaluated frequently. An ultrasound or CT can be helpful, but cannot exclude some important injuries. Peritoneal lavage may be used to assess whether there is any internal bleeding, but the results should be interpreted with care.

Liver trauma
Background
This is usually associated with other severe injuries.

Clinical presentation
A diagnosis of liver trauma is suspected if the patient is hypovolaemic and there is bruising or fracture of overlying ribs.

Management
A CT scan is useful for assessing the liver. Subcapsular or intrahepatic haematomas are treated conservatively. If there is major liver disruption then an urgent laparotomy to pack or resect the liver is needed.

Splenic rupture
Background
This can occur after minor trauma to a diseased spleen.

Clinical presentation
The presence of left shouldertip pain, hypovolaemia, and abdominal distension, and fractures of ribs 9–11 should suggest this diagnosis.

Management
A ruptured spleen is removed, but in children efforts are made to conserve it because of its important immunological functions.

Renal tract trauma
Clinical presentation
A suspicion of renal tract trauma is aroused if the patient has haematuria and fractured lower ribs or a lumbar spine injury. If the kidney is avulsed the patient is hypovolaemic and there is a flank haematoma, but no haematuria.

Management
Urgent nephrectomy is usually indicated for an avulsed kidney. A renal haematoma causes haematuria and usually resolves spontaneously.

Bladder rupture presents as peritonitis.

Urethral damage occurs in men who have a pelvic fracture or perineal trauma. There will be perineal bruising and the prostate will lie high. If it is suspected a urethrogram is performed before catheter insertion.

HEAD INJURY

Background
Direct or decelerating trauma damages the skull and brain:
- Primary brain damage is directly related to the trauma.
- Secondary brain damage occurs as a result of hypoxia, hypotension, infection, and intracranial bleeding.

Clinical presentation
In the conscious patient the following information should be obtained:
- Mechanism of the injury.
- Duration of time of loss of consciousness.
- Presence of headache, nausea, vomiting, blurred vision, dizziness, and retrograde amnesia.

Note that many of these patients, however, are influenced by the effects of alcohol and drugs.

Management
All patients should be evaluated using:
- The Glasgow coma scale (see Chapter 22, Fig. 22.10).
- Other observations including blood pressure, pulse, respiration, pupillary response, bruising, and presence of rhinorrhoea or otorrhoea.
- Assessment of the tone, power, and sensation of the limbs.

Careful examination is made for other injuries. Patients should be carefully and frequently re-evaluated to detect change.

Patients should be resuscitated to prevent secondary brain damage from hypoxia and may require intubation and ventilation.

A skull radiograph is obtained if there has been blunt or penetrating or open injury and a computed tomography (CT) scan is performed if the patient is unconscious or intracranial pathology is suspected.

Fig. 40.5 shows the signs of deterioration following to a head injury.

Skull fractures
Background
It is possible to have a fracture, but no intracranial pathology and vice versa.

Management
No action is necessary for a simple linear fracture unless there is intracranial damage. If there is a depressed fracture that is depressed more than the thickness of the skull operative elevation is required to prevent scarring to the brain and a risk of epilepsy.

Signs of deterioration following a head injury

Glasgow coma score decrease >2
headache, nausea, vomiting
↑ blood pressure; ↓ heart and respiratory rate
  (i.e. ↑ intracranial pressure)
↓ conscious level
↑ size of one or both pupils
weakness

Fig. 40.5 Signs of deterioration following a head injury.

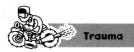

Compound fractures need early operative intervention, antibiotics, and skin closure to prevent infection.

Basal skull fractures are not evident on skull radiographs, but are suspected if there is cerebrospinal fluid rhinorrhoea or otorrhoea or Battle's sign (i.e. ecchymoses of the mastoid area, haemotympanum, and periorbital bruising). Management is conservative with antibiotics to prevent infection.

A frontal fracture is suspected if the patient has a subconjunctival haemorrhage and the posterior limit is not visible. The patient may also have anosmia or rhinorrhoea.

Acute cerebral injury
Background
A focal injury may be due to a haematoma or contusion.

Acute extradural haematoma
Acute extradural haematoma (Fig. 40.6) usually follows a fall or assault. It is due to a tear in a dural artery (e.g. middle meningeal artery) and is associated with a fracture in the temperoparietal region.

Clinical presentation
The features of acute extradural haematoma are:
- Initial loss of consciousness followed by a lucid interval and later loss of consciousness.

- Dilated and fixed ipsilateral pupil—due to stretching of the oculomotor nerve (3rd cranial nerve).
- Contralateral hemiparesis.
- Signs of increased intracranial pressure.

Management
An urgent CT scan and evacuation of clot via a burr hole are necessary.

Acute subdural haematoma
Background
Acute subdural haematoma (see Fig. 40.6) is due to the rupture of the veins bridging the space between the arachnoid mater and the dura mater.

Clinical presentation
There may not be an associated skull fracture, but there is often underlying brain injury.

Management
Emergency evacuation is required, but there is a high mortality rate.

Chronic subdural haematoma
Background
A trivial injury in the elderly may go unnoticed, but it may tear a vein between the arachnoid and dura mater.

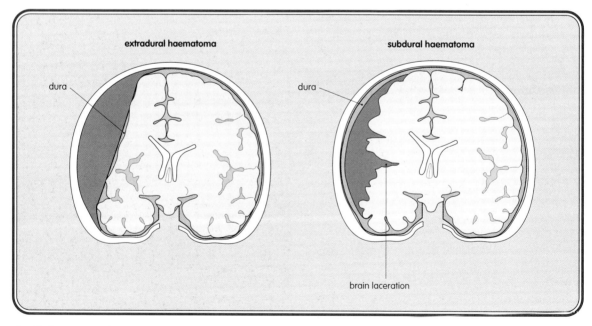

Fig. 40.6 Location of extradural and subdural haematomas.

Clinical presentation

A haematoma slowly enlarges by absorption of cerebrospinal fluid. There is a slow neurological deterioration with drowsiness, headache, and hemiplegia.

Management

Treatment is by evacuation.

Intracerebral haematoma

The neurological signs of intracerebral haematoma depend upon the area of brain affected. It is diagnosed by CT scan and management is conservative.

Diffuse brain injury

Diffuse brain injury is more common than a localized haematoma after a vehicle accident. Rapid head motion with acceleration and deceleration forces causing coup and contrecoup injuries. This causes diffuse axonal injury, cerebral oedema, and diffuse microscopic damage throughout the brain.

The patient is unconscious and full supportive treatment is given while awaiting improvement.

If the patient has a brain stem injury he or she is comatose and may have a decerebrate or decorticate posture. There is associated autonomic dysfunction with a high fever, hypertension, and sweating.

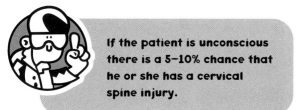

If the patient is unconscious there is a 5–10% chance that he or she has a cervical spine injury.

LIMB INJURIES

Clinical presentation

Limb injuries are very common. The bones may be fractured and joints dislocated. The injury may be compound or may be associated with vascular (Fig. 40.7) or neurological injury.

Management

Assessment includes examination to check the pulses and detect any neurological or functional deficit and any soft tissue injuries.

Any dislocation is reduced, the circulation is restored, fractures are immobilized, and soft tissue injuries are debrided.

BURNS

Management

The assessment of any patient who has burns includes a full history and examination looking for signs of smoke inhalation or thermal injury, which may cause oedema of the airway and may necessitate intubation. Blood gases should be measured.

The area affected is assessed using the 'rule of nines' (Fig. 40.8) and the thickness of the burns is assessed as:

Signs of vascular injury

haemorrhage
expanding haematoma
abnormal or absent pulses
impaired distal circulation
decreased sensation
increasing pain

Fig. 40.7 Signs of vascular injury.

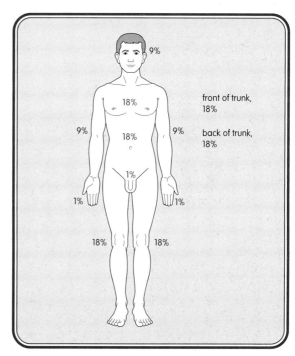

Fig. 40.8 'Rule of nines' for estimating area burned.

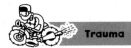

- First degree or superficial—may be due to a scald and characterized by erythema, blisters, and sensitivity to pinprick. This heals with normal skin within 14 days.
- Second degree or partial thickness—caused by scalds, contact, or flame burns of thick skin. The lesions are pink with white areas that have dull pinprick sensation. These heal within 3–4 weeks, but with poor quality skin and hypertrophic scars.
- Third degree or full thickness—caused by chemicals, flames, contact burns, or scalds. These burns appear dark and leathery and are painless. They can only heal by epithelialization from the edges, so form contracted scars.

The raw surface of burns loses a large quantity of fluid in the first 24–48 hours so adequate resuscitation is vital, for burns of more than 15% of body surface area (BSA).

The fluid requirement with colloid solution is calculated as:

Volume of fluid required (mL/unit time = [Total percentage of burn $\times$ weight (kg)]/2 for the first four 4-hour periods and then 6-hourly

Patients who have burns are closely monitored for pulse, blood pressure, and urine output.

Simple wound dressings are sulphadiazine creams or povidone iodine solution to prevent infection.

Full-thickness burns need early skin grafting.

If the burns are extensive the patient is catabolic and requires nutritional support and strong analgesia.

The prognosis depends upon the extent of the burns, age of the patient, and other medical conditions. There is a 50% mortality rate for patients who have burns covering more than 50% BSA, and those who survive are faced with disabilities and multiple further operations.

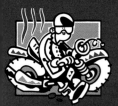

41. Postoperative Care and Complications

The postoperative period is very important for monitoring the patient to prevent immediate and long-term complications (Fig. 41.1). After the operation patients spend some time in the recovery ward where they are monitored until they are ready to return to the ward or high-dependency unit. Some patients who are seriously ill are transferred directly to the intensive care unit.

All of the patient's vital functions are monitored—airway, heart rate, blood pressure, conscious level, temperature (Fig. 41.2), respiratory rate and depth, oxygen saturation, and urine output, and the wound is assessed.

Complications are usually classified as:
- Immediate—within the first 24 hours.
- Early—occurring in the first 2–3 weeks postoperatively.
- Late— occurring at any subsequent period after discharge from hospital.
- General—affecting any of the body systems.
- Local—specific to the operation.

Complications of any operation are divided into those of any operation and those associated with a particular operation.

POSTOPERATIVE FLUID MANAGEMENT

Postoperative fluid requirements depend upon the type of operation performed and whether it is a maintenance or a replacement fluid regimen.

Normal homeostasis is maintained with 2–3 L/24 h of crystalloid fluid depending upon the age, weight of patient, and insensible losses.

Adequate fluid replacement is monitored by checking:
- Heart rate.
- Blood pressure.
- Urine output (which should be at least 0.5 mL/kg/h).

If the patient is very unwell and has cardiovascular impairment it may be helpful to insert a central venous pressure (CVP) line to monitor fluid replacement.

Maintenance requirements for 24 h is 1 L of normal saline and 2 L of 5% dextrose solution.

Potassium supplements are not necessary for 48 hours because antidiuretic hormone is secreted initially and there is retention of sodium and potassium. Subsequently at least 60 mmol of potassium chloride is necessary every 24 hours if the patient is on a minimal oral intake. If there are excess losses as a result of vomiting, fistula, or diarrhoea, the requirements are increased.

If there has been blood loss then it should be replaced. If the patient is actively bleeding colloid solutions can be used until blood is available. This stays in the circulation and draws extracellular fluid into the circulation by osmotic pressure so it is better than a crystalloid solution for maintaining blood pressure.

Colloid fluids are more effective than crystalloid fluids in maintaining blood pressure.

SHOCK

Background
Shock is defined as an inability to maintain adequate tissue perfusion and oxygenation. It may be:
- Hypovolaemic—inadequate circulatory volume due to haemorrhage or plasma losses or extracellular fluid depletion.
- Cardiogenic—the heart is unable to maintain cardiac output because of infarction or arrhythmia.
- Septicaemic—the presence of bacterial endotoxins causes peripheral vasodilatation and capillary permeability so the circulatory capacity is increased, but fluid leaks from the circulation.
- Anaphylactic—reaction to an antigen and as a result vasoactive substances cause vasodilatation and capillary permeability.

Clinical features and management of postoperative complications				
Complication	Time postoperatively	Cause	Signs and symptoms	Management
respiratory depression	<24 h	airway obstruction, GA or excess analgesia	↓ RR, ↓ conscious level, cyanosis	clear airway, reverse GA or effect of analgesia
hypovolaemia	<24 h	haemorrhage, inadequate fluid replacement, sepsis	↓ BP, ↑ HR, ↓ urine output	intravenous fluids—blood or colloids; antibiotics for sepsis
atelectasis	24–48 h	poor analgesia, smoking, previous chest problems	↑ temp., ↑ RR, ↓ O_2, ↓ AE bases of lungs	analgesia, physiotherapy, nebulizers
respiratory infection	>48 h	poor analgesia, smoking, previous chest problems	↑ temp., ↑ RR, ↓ O_2, ↓ AE and crepitations; sputum production	analgesia, physiotherapy, nebulizers and antibiotics
deep vein thrombosis (DVT)	5–10 days	operations causing immobility (e.g. pelvic, orthopaedic), oral contraceptive use, malignancy	↑ temp., leg swollen, tender calf	Doppler ultrasound or venogram; anticoagulation
pulmonary embolus (PE)	5–10 days	DVT, immobility, no signs of DVT in 50% of cases	present as pleuritic chest pains, multiple small PEs, or massive PE with collapse or death	ECG, V/Q scan, anticoagulation
wound infection	5 days	haematoma, contamination at operation, corticosteroid use, diabetes mellitus, malignancy, jaundice, long-duration operation	↑ temp. with red, tender and swollen wound	antibiotics
urinary tract infection	5 days	immobility, catheterization	↑ temp., confusion in elderly, dysuria	antibiotics ± drainage
wound dehiscence	5–10 days	poor operative technique, infection, haematoma, corticosteroid use	red serous discharge from wound, protruding intestine	resuscitation, return to theatre to repair wound
paralytic ileus	>4–5 days	normal response, but if occurs after >4–5 days there may be intra-abdominal pathology or ↓ K^+	NG aspirate, abdominal distension	resuscitation, NG aspiration, correct electrolytes
acute gastric dilatation	associated with paralytic ileus	vomiting, ↓ BP, ↑ HR	NG aspiration	
anastomotic dehiscence	5–10 days	poor operative technique, infection, diabetes mellitus, vascular insufficiency	↓ BP, ↑ temp., ↑ HR, peritonitis	resuscitation, laparotomy, antibiotics, lavage, defunction bowel
secondary haemorrhage	7–10 days	infection of suture line	↓ BP, ↑ HR, bleeding	resuscitation to stop haemorrhage
pseudomembranous colitis		following prolonged antibiotic use, due to *Clostridium difficile* toxin	diarrhoea, dehydration, abdominal pain	resuscitation, oral vancomycin

Fig. 41.1 Clinical features and management of postoperative complications. (AE, air entry; BP, blood pressure; ECG, electrocardiogram; GA, general anaesthetic; HR, heart rate; K^+, potassium ions; O_2, oxygen; NG, nasogastric; temp., temperature; RR, respiratory rate; V/Q scan, ventilation/perfusion scan.)

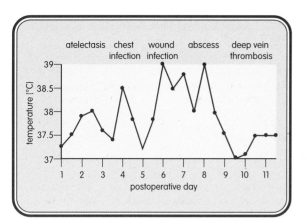

Fig. 41.2 Postoperative temperature chart showing possible causes of a postoperative pyrexia with the average time of onset in days.

Clinical presentation
Clinical features of shock are:
- Weak, rapid pulse.
- Hypotension.
- Hypoxia.
- Confusion.
- Decreased urine output.

In the initial stages of septic shock the peripheries may be warm and the patient may have a bounding pulse resulting from a hyperdynamic circulation.

Whatever the original cause the patient needs intensive monitoring and treatment to improve tissue perfusion and oxygenation to prevent further complications.

The main treatments are:
- Oxygenation.
- Fluid replacement.
- Treatment of sepsis.
- Control of arrhythmias.
- Use of inotropes to improve cardiac and renal function.

Complications of shock
Shock may precipitate acute respiratory distress syndrome (ARDS), acute renal failure, disseminated intravascular coagulation (DIC), acute hepatic failure, and stress ulceration. Patients may then develop systemic inflammatory response syndrome (SIRS), which may progress to multiorgan failure (MOF).

Each organ that is failing carries a mortality rate of 30%.

Acute respiratory distress syndrome
This is often precipitated by trauma, chest injury, sepsis, and pancreatitis. As part of sepsis toxins damage the endothelium of the lung capillaries—the lungs become oedematous and fibrin and microaggregates collect in the interstitial spaces so gas transfer is affected and the oxygen saturation decreases. A chest radiograph shows diffuse pulmonary infiltrates. Treatment is ventilation and supportive measures.

Acute renal failure
This is usually secondary to hypovolaemia or sepsis, which cause acute tubular necrosis (ATN). The urine output is less than 20 mL/h and the urea and potassium then start to increase.

The patient is dialysed until the kidney recovers, which should take 1–3 weeks if the acute renal failure is due to ATN. This is evident by a diuretic phase and the production of unconcentrated urine.

Disseminated intravascular coagulation
In sepsis the clotting factors are activated so widespread intravascular clotting occurs and then spontaneous haemorrhage. The diagnosis is confirmed by the presence of high levels of fibrin degradation products (FDPs).

Treatment of DIC is intravenous heparin to prevent clotting and normal clotting factors are given.

PREVENTION OF COMPLICATIONS

Antibiotic prophylaxis
The risk of infection depends upon the operation performed. Wounds are defined as:
- Clean—the mucosal surfaces are not breached and there is no local infection.
- Potentially contaminated—the mucosal surfaces are breached and exposed (e.g. elective gastrointestinal operation).
- Contaminated—there is established local infection or tissue soiling (e.g. peritonitis).

Prophylactic antibiotics are used to prevent infection from transient bacteraemia. The antibiotics used should have a broad spectrum of action and be bactericidal. They are given 1 hour before the transient bacteraemia so there is a high tissue level at the appropriate time. Usually 2–3 doses are given in 24 hours.

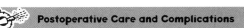
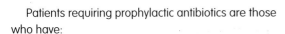
Patients requiring prophylactic antibiotics are those who have:

- Potentially contaminated operations or instrumentation of an infected site (e.g. endoscopic retrograde cholangiopancreatography for bile duct stones).
- Damaged or prosthetic valves or who have a prosthesis (e.g. hip prosthesis).

Prophylactic antibiotics should therefore be given for all gastrointestinal, genitourinary, and vascular (risk of causing gas gangrene) operations, and orthopaedic operations when a prosthesis is inserted.

Prophylactic antibiotics should be given if any prosthesis is present or to be inserted.

Prevention of deep vein thrombosis

Surgical operations predispose to deep vein thrombosis (DVT) because postoperatively the clotting factors and the number and stickiness of the platelets increase. During the operation the limbs are immobilized and the muscle pump does not function so there is stasis in the veins.

Risk factors for the development of DVT are:
- Age—over 40 years of age.
- Oral contraceptive use.
- Obesity.
- Diabetes mellitus.
- Polycythaemia.
- Varicose veins.

An increased risk for developing DVT is associated with:
- Operations for malignancy.
- Pelvic operations.
- Orthopaedic operations on the lower limbs.

Prevention of DVT is by use of thromboembolic compression stockings, administration of subcutaneous calcium heparin, and use of pneumatic calf compression intraoperatively.

POSTOPERATIVE ANALGESIA

It is very important to make sure that patients are free from pain postoperatively so that they can avoid some of the complications associated with immobility such as:
- Respiratory infection.
- DVT.
- Pressure sores.
- Urinary retention.

Patients who are prepared preoperatively have reduced postoperative anxiety and analgesic needs. The strength of the analgesia and its mode of administration depends upon the type of operation:

- Major abdominal or thoracic operations require opiates, which can be given continuously intravenously or using a patient-controlled analgesia (PCA) system. Alternative routes are epidural or intramuscular injections, but these give poor control due to erratic absorption.
- Pain of minor surgery can be controlled by the use of simple analgesics or non-steroidal anti-inflammatory drugs (NSAIDs), which can be given orally or rectally. Nerve blocks or infiltration of the wound with local anaesthetic are beneficial.

POSTOPERATIVE NUTRITION

Many patients undergoing gastrointestinal operations are malnourished preoperatively and have an increased risk of postoperative morbidity and death because of:
- Decreased resistance to infection.
- Impaired wound healing.

A history of recent weight loss is suggestive of malnutrition. Preoperative feeding may be of benefit to selected patients.

If patients are malnourished or experience complications of the operation so they cannot resume eating within a few days they should be fed. It is better to feed enterally because the integrity of the gut mucosal barrier and secretion of gut hormones and enzymes is maintained. The feed is given via a fine-bore nasogastric tube or gastrostomy or jejunostomy tube.

If gastrointestinal function is satisfactory the feed can be a complete polymeric feed, but if the digestive enzymes are inadequate an elemental feed is given.

Total parenteral nutrition (TPN) should be given via a CVP line to some patients who have a short gut, pancreatitis, or a high-output fistula. Possible complications are:

- Vascular damage.
- Haemopericardium.
- Haemopneumothorax.
- Thrombosis.
- Line sepsis.

The nutritional effects need to be closely monitored.

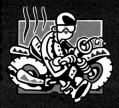

42. Principles of Cancer Management

CANCER

Cancer accounts for 1 in 4 deaths in the UK. It is the uncontrolled proliferation of abnormal cells. Tumour cells dedifferentiate so they become less like the parent cells and their growth is no longer inhibited by contact with neighbouring cells, but they have the capacity to invade and destroy adjacent normal structures—the lymphatic and venous channels.

Tumour size depends upon the cell cycle time, growth fraction, and the number of cells lost from the tumour surface. For a tumour to be palpable there are at least 10^9 cells and in most cases more.

Factors affecting the prognosis of cancer are:
- **Histological type**
- **Size of tumour**
- **Stage at presentation**
- **Age of patient**
- **Treatment available**

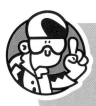

A simple classification of tumours is benign or malignant, primary or secondary.

Background

Most cancers are idiopathic, but there are some direct causal relationships:
- Smoking and lung cancer.
- Chemical exposure in the dye industry and bladder cancer.
- Ultraviolet radiation and skin cancer.
- Genetic abnormality resulting in familial polyposis coli and colon cancer.

Clinical presentation

There are several presentations of malignant disease:
- Specific symptom related to a localized cancer (e.g. breast cancer, skin cancer).
- Symptoms caused by the primary cancer (e.g. haemoptysis and lung cancer or rectal bleeding and rectal cancer).
- Systemic symptoms caused by the cancer (e.g. anaemia due to gastric cancer).
- Systemic symptoms related to ectopic hormone production (e.g. ectopic adrenocorticotrophic hormone production).
- Symptoms of metastatic disease (e.g. jaundice from liver secondaries or bone pain from bone metastases).

General features of advanced malignancy include malaise and weight loss, but it is hoped that most patients present before these systemic signs develop when the cancer is more likely to be treatable and curable.

Other syndromes related to malignancy are:
- Ectopic antidiuretic hormone secretion causing hyponatraemia.
- Neurological syndromes.
- Skin lesions such as dermatomyositis and acanthosis nigrans.

SCREENING FOR CANCER

This is the process of investigating an asymptomatic population that is at risk of a disease. The aim is to decrease the mortality rate from the disease. For screening to be effective the disease must have:
- A high population incidence.
- A detectable presymptomatic stage.

The test needs to be acceptable, cheap, reproducible, sensitive, and specific to the disease. Once detected there should be treatment available. For screening to be cost-effective there should be high compliance by the population at risk.

In the UK there are national screening programmes for breast cancer and cervical cancer. Recommended regimens for screening are:

- Breast cancer—50–64-year-old women —3-yearly bilateral mammograms.
- Cervical cancer—20–64-year-old women —5-yearly cervical smears.

Screening for colorectal cancer is only offered to those who have an increased risk because faecal occult blood testing is less acceptable to patients and colonoscopy is highly labour intensive.

Screening for early gastric cancer by barium meal and gastroscopy is carried out in Japan.

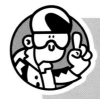

Epithelial cancers spread via the lymphatics and bloodstream, sarcomas spread via the bloodstream.

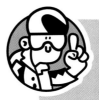

Complications of malignancy may be local, metastatic, or systemic (including paraneoplastic syndromes).

SPREAD OF CANCER

Invasive cancer means that the basement membrane has been breached and that the tumour is capable of spreading into the adjacent tissues, especially the lymphatics and venous channels so the cells can be transported to other fertile sites to form a secondary metastasis. The cells adhere to the vascular endothelium and the basement membrane is digested by the release of enzymes such as collagenase, which facilitates invasion of the tissue parenchyma. Fig. 42.1 shows the routes of cancer spread.

STAGING OF CANCER

The extent and degree of malignancy of a tumour are defined clinically and pathologically. This helps to plan treatment and gives an indication of the prognosis.

Pathological staging is based on the TNM classification (i.e. the extent of the tumour, nodes, and metastases).

Further tests such as blood tests for tumour markers and imaging by chest radiograph, computed tomography (CT) scan, and bone scan may be required to assess the patient.

Fig. 42.1 Routes of cancer spread.

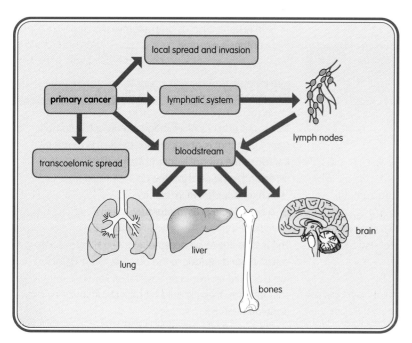

Histological grading refers to:
- Degree of differentiation of the tumour.
- Degree of nuclear polymorphism.
- Mitotic rate.

Treatment depends upon the stage of the disease. There is often a multidisciplinary approach, which uses a combination of surgery, chemotherapy, radiotherapy, or hormonal treatment. Different forms of treatment may be appropriate at different time periods of the disease (e.g. mastectomy for breast cancer and radiotherapy 10 years later for a bone secondary).

OPERATIONS FOR MALIGNANT DISEASE

Operations may be required at different times in the disease process. The main types of operation are:
- Diagnostic biopsies—for example lymph node biopsy to diagnose lymphoma.
- Primary excision—excision of the primary lesion with a margin of normal tissue in the longitudinal and lateral directions. This is usually combined with excision of the blood supply and the associated lymphatic drainage and nodes.
- Palliative surgery—it may not be possible to excise the primary tumour because of its invasion into vital structures, but operation may be performed to relieve symptoms (e.g. gastroenterostomy for antral gastric cancer or defunctioning colostomy for inoperable rectal cancer). Surgical excision may be appropriate even if metastases are present (e.g. mastectomy for a fungating breast cancer).
- Reconstructive surgery—after radical resection of some tumours the defect may need a reconstructive operation (e.g. pectoralis major flap after a head and neck operation or a rectus abdominis flap for breast reconstruction).

RADIOTHERAPY FOR MALIGNANT DISEASE

Tissues vary in their sensitivity to radiotherapy, for example squamous cell carcinomas are more sensitive than adenocarcinomas. There are several indications for its use:

- Primary treatment—for some skin cancers, carcinoma of the larynx, or squamous cell carcinoma of the oesophagus.
- Preoperative—to decrease the tumour mass.
- Postoperative adjuvant treatment after excision of primary tumour—to decrease the chance of local recurrence.
- Palliative for bone metastases, superior vena caval obstruction, or spinal cord compression.
- Systemic treatment—whole body irradiation of leukaemic patients having a bone marrow transplant.

Mechanism of action of radiotherapy

External beam radiotherapy from a linear accelerator produces high-energy X-rays, which interact with the molecules of the body tissues to cause ionization and release high-energy electrons, which cause secondary damage to adjacent molecules, including DNA via oxygen-dependent reactions. Large tumours are therefore more difficult to treat because hypoxic areas are more resistant to radiotherapy.

Some of the DNA damage cannot be repaired, resulting in chromosomal abnormalities, which prevent normal mitoses of cells so they die when they try to divide. Tumour cells are no more sensitive than normal cells to DNA damage, but are less able to repair it.

The dose of radiotherapy given is careful balanced to damage malignant cells while avoiding damage to normal tissues. The dose is fractionated to allow normal cells time to recover. Before radiotherapy is carried out there is careful planning of the fields so that the maximum dose is given to the smallest volume of tissue.

Complications of radiotherapy

These are usually due to the effect of radiotherapy on normal tissues. The sensitivity to damage and its expression depends upon the differing proliferation characteristics of each tissue. Early effects on different tissues include the following:
- Skin—desquamation.
- Mucosa of upper gastrointestinal tract—mucositis, oesophagitis.
- Intestine—vomiting, diarrhoea, ulceration, bleeding.
- Bladder—cystitis.

Tissues affected by late effects of radiotherapy include:
- Gonads—infertility.
- Thyroid gland—hypothyroidism.

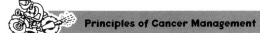

- Bowel—strictures due to impaired vascularity and fibrosis.
- Heart—ischaemic heart disease.
- Lymphatics—lymphoedema.

CHEMOTHERAPY FOR MALIGNANT DISEASE

The aim of chemotherapy is to selectively destroy malignant cells while sparing the normal cells, but the drugs interfere with the cell division of both normal and abnormal cells. The rate of proliferation of tumour cells varies in the tumour's life-time:

- In the early stages of tumour growth the growth fraction is high.
- As the tumour enlarges the growth fraction is low as the growth rate slows.

Chemotherapy is therefore less effective for larger tumours. The chemotherapy kills a constant fraction of the cells not a constant number.

There are four groups of chemotherapeutic agents:

- Alkylating agents.
- Antimetabolites.
- Vinca alkaloids.
- Antimitotic antibiotics.

There are many different drugs and treatment schedules for different tumour types and the side effect profile is variable.

Role of chemotherapy

The role of chemotherapy differs from case to case and may be:

- Curative—it is the main form of treatment for lymphomas and leukaemias.
- Adjuvant—as an extra treatment for micrometastases after the main tumour has been surgically excised (e.g. breast cancer).
- Neoadjuvant or preoperative—to decrease the tumour mass before operation.

- Palliative—to delay progression and control symptoms of metastatic disease.

Complications of chemotherapy

The main complications of chemotherapy are:

- Metallic taste for 2–3 days.
- Bone marrow toxicity—causing anaemia, thrombocytopenia, decreased white cell count, and increased risk of infection.
- Mucositis.
- Nausea and vomiting—because of the effect on the chemoreceptor trigger zone.
- Diarrhoea—because of the effects on the rapidly dividing cells of the gastrointestinal tract
- Alopecia—occurs after 18–21 days with some drugs.

HORMONAL THERAPY FOR MALIGNANT DISEASE

Some tumours are hormone sensitive and therefore drugs that alter the hormone balance are effective as primary treatment or adjuvant treatment (e.g. the ovaries can be suppressed by luteinizing hormone releasing hormone (LHRH) superagonists—to treat breast cancer).

PALLIATIVE CARE

Many patients who have cancer reach a stage where cure is not possible and the aim of treatment is relief of symptoms to improve the quality of remaining life so that it is as comfortable and as meaningful as possible. The approach focuses on the whole patient and his or her family who are all coping with a mixture of emotions —anxiety, denial, anger, despair, depression, and fear.

Palliative care is a multidisciplinary team approach to provide psychological support and symptomatic control for the patient. Patients' main fears are uncontrollable pain and death. It is very important that communication is good and honest and that there are realistic targets and expectations at this difficult time.

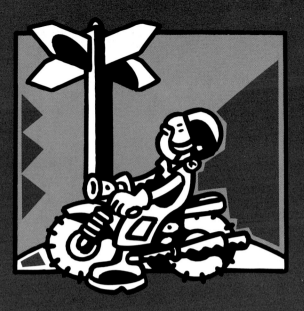

SELF-ASSESSMENT

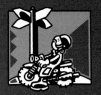

Multiple-choice Questions

Indicate whether each answer is true or false.

1. **Factors that increase the risk of a general anaesthetic include:**

a) Myocardial infarction over 2 years previously.
b) Gall stones.
c) Obesity.
d) Recent cerebrovascular accident.
e) Hypertension.

2. **The effects of smoking include:**

a) Increased activity of cilia.
b) Decreased immune function.
c) Decreased carbon monoxide concentration.
d) Increased risk of respiratory infection.
e) Negative inotropic effect.

3. **Examination of the hands may show:**

a) Clubbing associated with inflammatory bowel disease.
b) Koilonychia associated with liver disease
c) Dupuytren's contracture is due to fibrosis of the flexor tendons.
d) Palmar erythema, which is always a sign of liver disease.
e) Splinter haemorrhages associated with infective endocarditis.

4. **On examination of the abdomen:**

a) Murphy's sign is associated with acute appendicitis.
b) An enlarged spleen is always palpable.
c) 'Boardlike' rigidity is a sign of a perforated viscus.
d) A succussion splash is a sign of sigmoid volvulus.
e) A palpable gall bladder and jaundice is usually caused by gall stones.

5. **Concerning investigations before a general anaesthetic:**

a) All patients should have an electrocardiogram.
b) A macrocytic anaemia suggests chronic blood loss.
c) Patients who are on diuretics may develop hypokalaemia.
d) A low sodium level predisposes to arrhythmia.
e) Sickle cell test should be performed on Asian people.

6. **Concerning tumour markers:**

a) α-fetoprotein is a marker of ovarian cancer.
b) β-human chorionic gonadotrophin is a marker of testicular cancer and chorioncarcinoma.
c) CA125 is a marker of ovarian cancer.
d) Prostate-specific antigen is used routinely to screen for prostate cancer.
e) Carcinoembryonic antigen is a marker of recurrence of colon cancer.

7. **On a plain abdominal radiograph:**

a) Free gas may be seen in the peritoneal cavity.
b) 90% of gall stones are calcified.
c) Colonic dilatation is peripheral and the marks of the haustra are complete.
d) Loss of the psoas shadow implies retroperitoneal pathology.
e) Air in the biliary tree is a sign of a cholecystoduodenal fistula.

8. **Concerning oesophageal cancer:**

a) Presence of Barrett's oesophagus is a risk factor.
b) All oesophageal cancers are sensitive to radiotherapy.
c) Prognosis is good.
d) Most patients are treated by resection and colonic interposition.
e) Achalasia is a risk factor.

9. **About dysphagia:**

a) Achalasia usually presents in old age.
b) A double swallow is characteristic of achalasia.
c) Mitral stenosis can be a cause.
d) Reflux oesophagitis can cause a stricture.
e) Corkscrew oesophagus can be confused with myocardial ischaemia.

10. **Concerning peptic ulceration:**

a) It often occurs in association with *Helicobacter pylori* infection.
b) It can be treated with flucloxacillin and metronidazole.
c) Duodenal ulcer is associated with malignancy.
d) A duodenal ulcer is often treated by a highly selective vagotomy.
e) Recurrent ulceration may be a sign of a glucagonoma.

11. About gastric cancer:

a) Carcinoma of the cardia is decreasing in incidence.
b) Early gastric cancer is common in Japan.
c) Blood group O is a risk factor.
d) Most gastric cancers are squamous cell cancers.
e) It may be associated with Krukenberg's tumour.

12. Meckel's diverticulum:

a) Occurs in 20% of the population.
b) Is a common cause of rectal bleeding in children.
c) Can be diagnosed by a technetium pertechnetate scan.
d) May cause small bowel obstruction.
e) Is a pseudodiverticulum.

13. About Crohn's disease:

a) It only affects the small intestine.
b) Macroscopic appearance includes pseudopolyps and rose thorn ulcers.
c) Perianal problems may be the initial presentation.
d) Extraintestinal manifestations include arthritis and erythema nodosum.
e) It can be cured by a panproctocolectomy.

14. About small intestine tumours:

a) They are commonly malignant.
b) Carcinoid tumours of the appendix are usually asymptomatic.
c) They can be associated with skin pigmentation.
d) They may be familial.
e) Carcinoid syndrome only occurs if there are hepatic metastases.

15. Acute appendicitis:

a) Is a common diagnosis in children.
b) Usually resolves spontaneously.
c) Always produces rectal tenderness.
d) Often produces a pyrexia of 39°C.
e) Can cause dysuria and frequency.

16. About ulcerative colitis:

a) It may be associated with HLA B27.
b) It is usually treated with non-steroidal anti-inflammatory drugs.
c) Complications include perforation of the colon.
d) Microscopically there is full-thickness inflammation of the colon.
e) Kantor's string sign is a characteristic appearance on a barium enema.

17. Diverticulosis:

a) Is common in people under 35 years of age.
b) Is common in Africa.
c) May present with pneumaturia.
d) Usually occurs in the transverse colon.
e) Predisposes to colon cancer.

18. Concerning colonic cancer:

a) Risk factors include Crohn's disease and Gardener's syndrome.
b) Carcinoembryonic antigen is a reliable tumour marker.
c) 30% of tumours are synchronous.
d) The commonest site of colon cancer is the rectum.
e) Dukes' B cancer has spread to the lymph nodes.

19. Haemorrhoids:

a) Occur at the 2, 5, and 10 o'clock positions.
b) May be treated by an external sphincterotomy.
c) Are exacerbated by pregnancy.
d) If third degree, just bleed.
e) Injection sclerotherapy is painful.

20. About perianal abscess:

a) It may be related to an underlying fistula.
b) Staphylococcal infection is usually associated with a fistula.
c) It is a common presentation of ulcerative colitis.
d) It is common in diabetics.
e) A Seton suture is used to treat a high fistula and prevent incontinence.

21. Concerning ovarian cysts:

a) They always cause abdominal pain.
b) A 'chocolate cyst' is associated with endometriosis.
c) Dermoid cysts usually occur in women aged 40–50 years.
d) CA125 is a marker of ovarian cancer.
e) Chemotherapy has no role in the management of ovarian cancer.

22. About pelvic inflammatory disease:

a) It predisposes to an ectopic pregnancy.
b) Sexually transmitted pelvic inflammatory disease is usually caused by chlamydia.
c) It causes dyspareunia.
d) Hydrosalpinx is an obstructed fallopian tube containing pus.
e) Endometritis can occur postpartum.

23. Features of obstructive jaundice include:

a) Pruritus caused by bile pigments.
b) Increased alkaline phosphatase.
c) Prolonged clotting time.
d) Normal calibre bile ducts on ultrasound scan.
e) Risk of renal impairment.

24. Portal hypertension:

a) Develops if the portal pressure is over 5 mmHg.
b) Can be associated with schistosomiasis.
c) Can cause thrombocytopenia.
d) Predisposes to the development of rectal varices.
e) May be relieved by a transjugular intrahepatic shunt (TIPS).

25. About hepatic tumours:

a) Primary hepatocellular carcinoma is very common worldwide.
b) Carcinoembryonic antigen is associated with hepatoma.
c) Aflatoxins are a common cause of hepatoma.
d) Are associated with the use of the oral contraceptive.
e) Metastatic tumours are an unusual cause.

26. Concerning gall stones:

a) Over 10% are calcified.
b) Are common in patients with haemolytic disorders.
c) Charcot's triad is associated with acute cholecystitis.
d) Gall stones increase the risk of bleeding disorders.
e) They are associated with squamous cell cancer of the gall bladder.

27. About pancreatitis:

a) It can be due to hypocalcaemia.
b) Cullen's sign is bruising in the flank.
c) Calcium higher than 2 mmol/L is a feature of severe pancreatitis.
d) Oxygen less than 7.98 kPa is a feature of severe pancreatitis.
e) White cell count higher than 16×10^9/L is a feature of severe pancreatitis.

28. Concerning pancreatic tumours:

a) Most are benign.
b) Periampullary tumours can be treated by a pancreaticoduodenectomy.
c) Glucagonoma causes hypoglycaemia.
d) Zollinger–Ellison syndrome is associated with recurrent peptic ulceration.
e) Carcinoma is associated with thrombophlebitis migrans.

29. Inguinal hernia:

a) Appears above and lateral to the pubic tubercle.
b) Is common in children under 1 year of age.
c) Is uncommon in women.
d) If direct, is at risk of strangulation.
e) In adults it can be treated by a herniotomy.

30. Concerning other hernias:

a) A spigelian hernia is common.
b) A Richter's hernia is due to strangulation of part of the bowel.
c) Obturator hernia is common in men.
d) An obturator hernia produces pain down the lateral aspect of the thigh.
e) A sliding inguinal hernia often contains the caecum.

31. Signs of thyrotoxicosis include:

a) Dry skin.
b) Ophthalmoplegia.
c) Hoarse voice.
d) Periorbital puffiness.
e) Atrial fibrillation.

32. Diagnosis of thyrotoxicosis is confirmed by:

a) Increased thyroxine and increased thyroid stimulating hormone.
b) Presence of antimitochondrial antibodies.
c) Hot spot on a radioisotope scan.
d) Presence of long-acting thyroid stimulating antibodies.
e) Hypocalcaemia.

33. About thyroid cancers:

a) They usually occur in elderly people.
b) 60% of cases are papillary cancer.
c) Follicular cancer usually presents with pressure symptoms.
d) Lymphoma is related to Hashimoto's disease.
e) It can be diagnosed acccurately by fine-needle aspiration and cytology.

34. Potential complications of thyroid surgery include:

a) Hoarse voice.
b) Alteration of pitch of voice.
c) Hypercalcaemia.
d) Bovine cough.
e) Pyrexia, agitation, confusion.

35. Features of hyperparathyroidism include:

a) Hypocalcaemia and increased alkaline phosphatase.
b) Osteitis fibrosa cystica.
c) Bone pain.
d) Peptic ulceration.
e) Muscle spasms.

36. Concerning neck lumps:

a) Cervical lymphadenopathy may be due to nasopharyngeal cancer.
b) A branchial cyst is a midline structure.
c) A thyroglossal cyst usually presents in adults.
d) A branchial sinus discharges in the lower third of the neck.
e) Pleomorphic adenoma usually occurs in the submandibular glands.

37. About benign breast problems:

a) Mastalgia is often treated with bromocriptine.
b) Puerperal breast abscesses are usually due to coliforms.
c) Periductal mastitis is associated with smoking.
d) Cysts are associated with an increased risk of breast cancer.
e) Fibroadenomas are usually found in women under 30.

38. Concerning breast cancer:

a) Risk is increased if mother has cancer at 65 years of age.
b) Men who have breast cancer often have a family history of breast cancer.
c) It is associated with BRCA1 gene.
d) Over 25% of breast cancers are inherited.
e) Mortality rate is decreased by screening.

39. More questions on breast cancer:

a) Breast cancer is always seen on mammography.
b) Most breast cancers are invasive lobular cancers.
c) Ductal carcinoma in situ is the preinvasive stage of ductal cancer.
d) In the UK the breast screening programme is for women aged 45–65 years.
e) Paget's disease of the nipple affects the areola first.

40. Breast cancer treatment usually includes:

a) Adjuvant chemotherapy for premenopausal women.
b) Adjuvant chemotherapy for patients who are node positive and over 60 years of age.
c) Radiotherapy after local excision to decrease local recurrence.
d) Aminoglutethimide.
e) Oophorectomy for postmenopausal women.

41. Concerning abdominal aortic aneurysms:

a) They usually develop above the renal arteries.
b) They may be confused with ureteric colic.
c) They can cause congestive cardiac failure and lower limb ischaemia.
d) A complication of the repair is colonic ischaemia.
e) Elective surgical repair has an 85% mortality rate.

42. Neuropathic ulcers are associated with:

a) Good peripheral pulses.
b) Cold feet.
c) Diabetes mellitus.
d) Charcot's joints.
e) Pain.

43. Ischaemic changes in the hands may be due to:

a) Cervical rib.
b) Thromboangiitis obliterans.
c) Lipodermatosclerosis.
d) Thrombophlebitis.
e) CREST syndrome.

44. Complications of urinary tract infection include:

a) Renal failure.
b) Hydronephrosis.
c) Staghorn calculus.
d) Xanthogranulomatous pyelonephritis.
e) Hypernephroma.

45. Concerning malignancy of the genitourinary tract:

a) Pyrexia of unknown origin may be a sign of a hypernephroma.
b) Nephroblastoma is associated with a poor prognosis.
c) Bladder tumours are usually squamous cell carcinomas.
d) Bladder cancer is associated with the dye industry.
e) Bladder cancer usually presents with painful haematuria.

46. Prostate cancer:

a) Arises in the periphery of the gland.
b) If graded as T4 is confined to the gland.
c) Is hormone independent.
d) Can be detected reliably by measuring prostate-specific antigen.
e) Causes sclerotic deposits.

47. Obstruction of the upper urinary tract:

a) Can be relieved by catheterization.
b) May cause pyonephrosis.
c) May be due to retroperitoneal fibrosis.
d) Is rarely caused by pelviureteric obstruction.
e) Can cause acute retention.

48. Concerning testicular problems:

a) An operation for undescended testis should be performed after 5 years of age.
b) Orchidopexy is excision of the testis
c) Testicular torsion usually occurs in adolescent boys.
d) Teratoma is a condition of old men.
e) Torsion can present with abdominal pain and vomiting.

49. The following are premalignant skin lesions:

a) Dermatofibroma.
b) Keratoacanthoma.
c) Bowen's disease.
d) Solar keratoses.
e) Rodent ulcer.

50. Signs of raised intracranial pressure include:

a) Decreased blood pressure.
b) Decreased heart rate.
c) Fixed dilated pupil.
d) Decrease in Glasgow Coma Scale score.
e) Increased respiratory rate.

1. What are the symptoms and complications of a rolling hiatus hernia?

2. What are the common causes of dysphagia in an elderly person? How would you investigate the patient?

3. What are the potential complications of a hernia? Which types of hernia are most likely to cause problems?

4. What are the clinical features of obstructive jaundice? How would you plan the investigations?

5. What precautions should be taken before intervention in any patient with jaundice?

6. List the common causes of obstructive jaundice?

7. What are the possible complications of diverticulosis?

8. List the pathological and radiographic features of Crohn's disease?

9. What is meant by triple assessment of a breast lump?

10. Describe the clinical features of a fibroadenoma, cyst and cancer?

11. What are the features of intermittent claudication and rest pain? What is their significance?

12. List the clinical features and causes of an acutely ischaemic limb?

13. Why do diabetics have an increased risk of developing foot ulcers?

14. What are the causes of a solitary thyroid nodule? Outline the management plan for this problem?

15. What are the possible causes of upper urinary tract obstruction in an adult? Outline the management of this problem?

16. What are the possible complications of urinary tract infection?

17. What observations should be made after a general anaesthetic?

18. What are the common postoperative chest complications?

19. What are the possible causes of a pyrexia 5 days after a colonic resection?

20. What is the Glasgow Coma Scale and what is its significance?

1. A 23-year-old woman presents with a 12-hour history of lower abdominal pain.

   a) Outline the other information you would obtain from the history.
   b) What is your differential diagnosis?
   c) What tests could you do as an emergency?

2. A 56-year-old man presents with sudden onset of generalized abdominal pain.

   a) Outline your plan of emergency management.
   b) His amylase result is 1500 IU/L. What additional investigations would you perform to assess the severity of the attack?

3. A 75-year-old man presents to his general practitioner complaining of a change of bowel habit over the last few months.

   a) What is your differential diagnosis?
   b) How would you investigate him?
   c) A barium enema shows a sigmoid carcinoma. What is the likely treatment?
   d) How would you counsell this man prior to surgery?

4. An 82-year-old man presents with a short history of progressive dysphagia.

   a) What features of the history may give you a clue to the likely cause?.
   b) How would you manage this man and what is the likely prognosis?

5. A 74-year-old lady is admitted as an emergency with a 3-hour history of sudden onset of profuse dark red rectal bleeding. On admission she is pale with a pulse of 100/min and a blood pressure of 100/60 mmHg.

   a) What are the possible causes of this scenario?

6. At the breast clinic a 48-year-old lady presents because she has noticed an irregular non-tender lump in the upper outer aspect of her right breast.

   a) Describe how this lady will be assessed?
   b) The tests show that this is a breast carcinoma. Outline the treatment options for this woman, including any adjuvant treatment.

7. A 63-year-old lady presents with a history of obstructive jaundice. She has a past history of biliary colic.

   a) How would you investigate and treat this lady?
   b) What precautions would you take before any surgical intervention?

8. A 57-year-old lady presents to her general practitioner with a history of lethargy, shortness of breath and angina. After initial examination the general practitioner thinks that she looks anaemic.

   a) How would you proceed with further investigations?
   b) What are the possible causes of this lady's anaemia?

9. A 65-year-old man complains of painless macroscopic haematuria of recent onset?

   a) How would you investigate him?
   b) A cystoscopy shows a bladder cancer. How would you stage it and plan treatment?

10. An 83-year-old man has a history of intermittent claudication and presents with a 3-hour history of a cold painful leg.

    a) What is the likely underlying cause?
    b) How would you manage the situation?

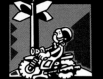

MCQ Answers

1. a) F, b) F, c) T, d) T, e) T
2. a) F, b) T, c) F, d) T, e) T
3. a) T, b) F, c) F, d) F, e) T
4. a) F, b) F, c) T, d) F, e) F
5. a) F, b) F, c) T, d) F, e) T
6. a) F, b) T, c) T, d) F, e) T
7. a) T, b) F, c) F, d) T, e) T
8. a) T, b) F, c) F, d) F, e) T
9. a) F, b) F, c) T, d) T, e) T
10. a) T, b) F, c) F, d) F, e) F
11. a) F, b) T, c) F, d) F, e) T
12. a) F, b) T, c) T, d) T, e) F
13. a) F, b) F, c) T, d) T, e) F
14. a) F, b) T, c) T, d) T, e) T
15. a) T, b) F, c) F, d) F, e) T
16. a) T, b) F, c) T, d) F, e) F
17. a) F, b) F, c) T, d) F, e) F
18. a) F, b) T, c) F, d) T, e) F
19. a) F, b) F, c) T, d) F, e) F
20. a) T, b) F, c) F, d) T, e) T
21. a) F, b) T, c) F, d) T, e) F
22. a) T, b) T, c) T, d) F, e) T
23. a) F, b) T, c) T, d) F, e) T
24. a) F, b) T, c) T, d) T, e) T
25. a) T, b) F, c) T, d) T, e) F

26. a) F, b) T, c) F, d) F, e) F
27. a) F, b) F, c) F, d) T, e) T
28. a) F, b) T, c) F, d) T, e) T
29. a) F, b) T, c) T, d) F, e) F
30. a) F, b) T, c) F, d) F, e) F
31. a) F, b) T, c) F, d) F, e) T
32. a) F, b) F, c) T, d) T, e) F
33. a) F, b) T, c) F, d) T, e) F
34. a) T, b) T, c) F, d) T, e) T
35. a) F, b) T, c) T, d) T, e) F
36. a) T, b) F, c) F, d) T, e) F
37. a) F, b) F, c) T, d) F, e) T
38. a) F, b) T, c) T, d) F, e) F
39. a) F, b) F, c) T, d) F, e) F
40. a) T, b) F, c) T, d) F, e) F
41. a) F, b) T, c) T, d) T, e) F
42. a) T, b) F, c) T, d) T, e) F
43. a) T, b) T, c) F, d) F, e) T
44. a) T, b) F, c) T, d) T, e) F
45. a) T, b) F, c) F, d) T, e) F
46. a) T, b) F, c) F, d) F, e) T
47. a) F, b) T, c) T, d) F, e) F
48. a) F, b) F, c) T, d) F, e) T
49. a) F, b) F, c) T, d) T, e) F
50. a) F, b) T, c) T, d) T, e) F

SAQ Answers

1. The symptoms may be those of gastro-oesophageal reflux with the addition of intermittent dysphagia, cardiac symptoms, and hiccoughs due to phrenic nerve irritation.

   The complications may include peptic ulceration and incarceration, which may cause strangulation and ischaemia. It may be a cause of a gastric volvulus, which can become ischaemic and perforate causing sepsis in the thorax or peritoneal cavity.

2. The common causes of dysphagia in an elderly person are:
   - Benign peptic stricture with or without hiatus hernia.
   - Carcinoma of the oesophagus or gastric cardia.

   Less common causes are pharyngeal pouch, retrosternal goitre, enlarged hilar nodes, and neurological problems such as bulbar palsy.

   The investigations should include full blood count, and electrolytes if dehydrated or vomiting. The site and length of the obstruction is identified first by a barium swallow before a gastroscopy with or without biopsy because of the risk of perforation if endoscopy is not performed with care.

3. Most hernias are at risk of becoming irreducible and the contents of the sac may become strangulated and ischaemic, which can lead to perforation and sepsis. This often occurs to abdominal hernias and the small intestine is obstructed causing abdominal pain, vomiting and constipation.

   The feature of a hernia that predisposes to the development of complications is a narrow neck. This is a feature of an indirect inguinal hernia, femoral hernia, and paraumbilical hernia.

4. The clinical features of obstructive jaundice are:
   - Pale stools.
   - Dark urine.
   - Pruritus.

   Abdominal examination may reveal hepatomegaly or a palpable gall bladder if the obstruction is not due to gall stones. This may be associated with abdominal pain depending upon the underlying pathology.

   Initial investigations should include:
   - Blood tests for full blood count.
   - Electrolytes for renal function.
   - Liver function tests.
   - Clotting screen.
   - Hepatitis screen if there is a possibility of an infectious cause.
   - An ultrasound scan will show any dilated bile ducts and may show the level of obstruction and any possible causes such as gall stones, carcinoma of the pancreas or enlarged porta hepatis nodes.
   - A diagnostic and therapeutic endoscopic retrograde cholangiopancreatography following ultrasound scan if possible. If the patient has had a previous gastric operation it may be necessary to perform percutaneous transhepatic cholangiography instead to delineate the anatomy and insert a stent.
   - A computed tomography scan may be needed to stage a tumour.

5. Before any invasive procedure on a patient with obstructive jaundice precautions are taken to prevent the complications of:
   - Cholangitis and septicaemia.
   - Renal failure.
   - Disseminated intravascular coagulation.

   The patients should be well hydrated to maintain renal perfusion, any abnormal clotting is corrected with vitamin K and possibly clotting factors. Lactulose is given to prevent endotoxaemia and prophylactic antibiotics are administered to prevent bacteraemia and septicaemia.

6. The common causes of obstructive jaundice are:
   - Gall stones.
   - Pancreatic cancer.
   - Chronic pancreatitis.
   - Enlarged nodes in the porta hepatis.

   The less common causes are:
   - Cholangiocarcinoma.
   - Benign strictures of the biliary system.
   - Sclerosing cholangitis.
   - Gall bladder cancer.
   - Liver flukes.

7. Complications of diverticulosis include:
    - Diverticular stricture causing recurrent subacute obstruction.
    - Diverticulitis, which may resolve or form a paracolic abscess or perforate into the peritoneal cavity to cause peritonitis.
    - Formation of a vesicocolic fistula, which presents with pneumaturia and cystitis, or a colovaginal fistula, which causes a faeculent discharge per vaginum.
    - Haemorrhage from erosion of a vessel at the mouth of a diverticulum.

8. The macroscopic features of Crohn's disease are thickened oedematous red bowel with fat encroaching from the mesentery onto the bowel. There is 'cobblestone mucosa' and 'rose thorn' ulcers. Microscopically there is full-thickness inflammation with granulomas.
    Radiographic features include:
    - Skip lesions.
    - Kantor's string sign.
- Deep fissures.
- Signs of subacute obstruction (i.e. dilated loops of small intestine).

9. Triple assessment of a breast lump comprises:
    - Clinical examination and subsequent clinical impression.
    - Imaging by mammography or ultrasound examination
    - Cytology or histopathological assessment.

10. Fibroadenoma occurs in women aged 15–30 years. It is very mobile, smooth, well defined, and firm.
    A cyst usually occurs in women aged 30–50 years and may be tender. It is quite well defined, firm, and not very mobile. It may feel fluctuant and change in size with the menstrual cycle.
    Classically a breast cancer is hard and irregular, and may be associated with skin tethering or dimpling, deep fixation, nipple inversion, peau d'orange, or skin ulceration.

11. Intermittent claudication is a cramp-like pain that develops in the limb after exercise. It resolves after rest. It is a sign of ischaemia to the tissues and the pain is due to the accumulation of metabolites. In the long term it may improve if a collateral circulation develops and the patient stops smoking.
    Rest pain is a severe persistent pain that is a sign of critical ischaemia and impending irreversible tissue damage. The pain is worse at night if the limb is warm and therefore patients sleep in chairs so that the leg is dependent. It may be exacerbated by an infection or ulceration.

12. The features of an acutely ischaemic limb are:
    - Pulseless.
    - Painful.
    - Pallor.
    - Paraesthesia.
    - Paralysis.
    - Perishing cold.
    The common causes are an embolus secondary to atrial fibrillation or a myocardial infarction or thrombosis associated with atherosclerosis.

13. Diabetics have an increased risk of developing foot ulceration because of:
    - Peripheral neuropathy.
    - Atherosclerosis.
    - Microangiopathy.
    - Increased risk of infection because of hyperglycaemia.
    - Charcot's joints.

14. The differential diagnosis of a solitary thyroid nodule includes a thyroid cyst, benign thyroid adenoma, and thyroid malignancy.
    Investigation includes measurement of thyroid function tests and an ultrasound scan to differentiate between solid and cystic lumps. A radioisotope scan can differentiate between hot and cold nodules. Fine-needle aspiration and cytology is performed to differentiate benign from malignant cells, but cannot be used to differentiate well-differentiated cancers from benign lesions. If there is any doubt a thyroid lobectomy should be performed.

15. Common causes of upper urinary tract obstruction in adults are:
    - Pelviureteric junction obstruction.
    - Ureteric tumour.
    - Pelvic tumours (e.g. bladder, prostate, cervix or rectum).
    - Retroperitoneal fibrosis.
    - Radiation strictures.
    Diagnosis is made by ultrasound, which will demonstrate hydronephrosis. If the patient has acute renal failure he or she needs urgent dialysis and insertion of percutaneous nephrostomy tubes to decompress the kidney before definitive treatment for the obstruction.

16. Complications of urinary tract infection include:
    - Cystitis, prostatitis, and epididymo-orchitis.
    - Pyelonephritis, septicaemia, and perinephric abscess.
    - Chronic pyelonephritis, hypertension, and renal failure.
    - Xanthogranulomatous pyelonephritis.
    - Formation of staghorn calculi.

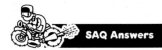

17. Postoperatively patients who have had a general
anaesthetic should be assessed for
- Conscious level.
- Respiratory depth and rate, oxygen saturation.
- Pulse rate and volume, blood pressure, urine output.
- Temperature.
- Wound and drainage.
- Pain control.

18. Common postoperative chest problems are:
- Respiratory depression due to anaesthesia or
analgesics—immediate and within 24 hours.
- Atelectasis—24–48 hours.
- Chest infection—after 48 hours.
- Pulmonary embolus—after 5 days.

19. Five days postoperatively a pyrexia may be due to:
- Chest or urinary tract infection.
- Deep vein thrombosis.
- Wound infection.
- Intra-abdominal abscess.
- Anastomotic dehiscence or peritonitis.

20. Glasgow Coma Scale assesses:
- Best motor response.
- Verbal response.
- Eye responses.

It is a reproducible assessment of conscious level so
that information can be recorded accurately and
passed on to other people.

A fully conscious patient has a score of 15; a score of
3 indicates the deepest level of coma. A score of less
than 8 indicates coma.

Index

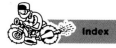

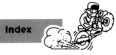

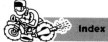